THE GLIMPSES
OF
THE HISTORY OF MEDICINE

THE GLIMPSES OF THE HISTORY OF MEDICINE

by

Dr. D. D. Banerjee M.B.S. (Homoeopathy)
Principal, P.C.M.H. Hospital & College
Member, Central Council for Homoeopathy

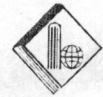

B. JAIN PUBLISHERS (P) LTD.
USA — EUROPE — INDIA

THE GLIMPSES OF THE HISTORY OF MEDICINE

7th Impression: 20*)

NOTE FROM THE PUBLISHERS
Any information given in this book is not intended to be taken as a replacement for medical advice. Any person with a condition requiring medical attention should consult a qualified practitioner or therapist.

All rights reserved. No part of this book may be reproduced, stored in a retrieval system or transmitted, in any form or by any means, mechanical, photocopying, recording or otherwise, without any prior written permission of the publisher.

© with the publisher

Published by Kuldeep Jain for
B. JAIN PUBLISHERS (P) LTD.
B. Jain House, D-157, Sector-63,
NOIDA-201307, U.P. (INDIA)
Tel.: +91-120-4933333 • *Email:* info@bjain.com
Website: www.bjain.com

Printed in India by
B B Press Noida

ISBN: 978-81-319-0350-6

ACKNOWLEDGEMENTS

1. *Studies in Arabic and Persian Medical Literature - by Prof. Muhammad Zubayr Siddiqui.*

2. *A History of Medicine - by Douglas Guthzie.*

3. *An Introduction to the History of Medicine - by Fielding H. Garrison.*

4. *History of Indian Medicine.*

PREFACE

Different academic councils and universities have given a chapter of the History of Medicine in their courses and curriculum for study. The History of Medicine of different countries from pre-historic era to twenty first century, may be treated as a specialised course and curriculum which may take several months to complete, which could not be possible for any under-graduate student, it is a matter of post-graduate study.

There are various books in diifferent languages in diifferent parts of the world. This is only an attempt to have an abridged one.

To the readers I apologize for any mistake, crept in due to printer's devil.

3, Chowringhee **D.D. Banerjee**
Calcutta

INTRODUCTION

The physician of to-day is the product of 20th and 21st Century revolutions in science and technology.

Appreciation of ultra molecular biology, genetical evolution and other forms of sophistication of different branches of science have come to such a stage, that the medical profession occasionally loses its relation to humanity.

Medicine is a life-long study and it is true that one must progressively acquire more and newer knowledge.

The pursuit of the truth of the laws of nature is defined as science. Man should try to understand himself and his surroundings and the evolution of scientific and technological progress.

A physician who does not wants to be dictated to by trade should be well conversant with the progress of science and try to realise man as a whole.

Technology can stagnate without the evolution of scientific progress. The present may be an evolutionary product or a disappointment of the past.

In March 1944 Sir Winston Churchill remarked that "The more you can look back, the further you can go forward."

The past bears the genesis of the present and future. History forms the basis of all knowledge and is the convenient avenue of approach to any subject or to any discipline of science.

As such it is natural to regard the evolution and progress of medicine from bygone times as an essential background to modern medical education.

The structure of the human society has radically altered during the last 200 years, spearheaded by Industrial revolution and end of feudalism.

We are trying for a new era, where the crude birth rate should be 21.0%, crude death rate 9.0%, annual growth rate 1.20%, rate of reproduction 1.0%, family size 2.3, effective couple protection rate 60%, infant mortality rate less than 60%, maternal mortality rate less than 2%.

Feudalistic ideas and beliefs were such that death comes as a punishment of man's disobedience to God are obsolete. The basic nature of human life, the forms, the patterns, intrinsic nature of ideas, beliefs, motives, the organisation and struggles of the society are heading for a newer patterns. Helmholt's conservation of Energy (1847), Darwin's origin of Species (1859), Virchow's cellular pathology (1858), Pavloff's science of conditional reflexes and researches in psychology including Psycho-somatic condition, did away forever with many silly propositions and gained importance in medicine.

Natural phenomena are being explained on a rational factional basis. Conception of health has taken a newer dimention.

The question of "the collective and individual" psychology and health has taken a foot-hold in the medical profession.

The Hippocratic tradition though it remained a living force for long years in the western world and tried to eliminate superstious and degenerating habits of life, yet could not give the right solution to the clinician.

It only pointed out that "Nature" should not be totally rejected. The clinicians went in serch of definite causative organism of ill health.

Different centres of learning at Indian sub-continent, China, Rome, Arabia, Egypt came up; universities like Bologna (1113 A.D.), Padua (1222 A.D.) were established for medical teaching. Previously it was religiously oriented. Gradually it was felt that the aim of medical education should be to produce a cultured and highly educated gentlemen or women with an adequate knowledge of medicine and unprejudiced observation for which one must have a minimum knowledge of historical background.

I have attempted to write a short synopsis of the history of medicine.

It is obivious that a work of this nature cannot be undertaken without assistance and I pay my gratitude to my friends specially to Dr. M. S. Zaman and Sri Somnath Chatterjee of Bishudhasram, Burdwan for their help.

I am also thankful to B.Jain Publishers (P) Ltd., Delhi for their co-operation.

6, *Kundu Road* **D.D. Banerjee**
Calcutta - 700025

14th November, 1988

CONTENTS

		Pages
1.	Pre Historic Era	1
2.	The first known Medical Personnel	4
3.	Egyptian Medicine	4
4.	Mohammedan and Jewish Period	10
5.	Medical culture of Mohammedans	11
6.	School of Salero	12
7.	12th and 13th Century (Mediaeval period)	14
8.	Restoration of Anatomy teaching	15
9.	Chinese	18
10.	Aphorisms and oath of Hippocratic	21
11.	15th and 16th Century Medicine	27
12.	16th Century - Paracelsus - Harvey	33
13.	17th Century - Boyle - Mayow Leeuwenhock	43 - 45
14.	18th Century Medicine	49
15.	19th Century and Renaissance period	52
16.	Radiology	92
17.	Psychiatry	95
18.	Anaesthetic Properties	103
19.	Antiseptics	107
20.	Catgut	111
21.	Gynaecology , Obstetric forcep' Opthalmology	113
22.	Bacteriology	123
23	Otology	130
24	Auscultation	135

Glimpses of History of Medicine

PRE HISTORIC ERA

The most difficult task in writing the history of any topic is the history of Medicine. It is very difficult to begin. In reality the history of medicine is related with the beginning of the mankind. Nothing documentary writing and evidences in respect of medical thought can be produced from the Storages of man, except certain drawings and specimens that have survived from the stone age. In those ages medical professional personnel were known as "Magicians". A drawing on the wall of the Trois Freres cave in Pyrenees is the potrait probably of an oldest medical man.

Numerous stones, and tools probably of 15,000 B.C. have been discovered, some of them may well have been employed as surgical instruments. The problem of death was thought as a punishment for man's disobedience. The existence of diseases was considered differently. Diseases were viewed as a result of malevolent influences exercised by a god or supernatural being or of another humanbeing alive or dead. As an example, it may be said that the aboriginals of Central Australia were still now considered to be the most primitive type of man. They have a peculiar custom of using a "Bone" made up by a long slender stick and was used to bring illness to a person by some ritual performance and songs, if fortunately the man becomes sick by any other influences, he used to go to a so-called "Magician Medicine Man" or a "priest" to get the evil influences sucked out and to take some indigenous herbs or used to take some methods of retaliation of the aggressors. But it will not be wise to undermine all their behaviours and knowledges because specimen of Trephining of skull evidently proves for their knowledge of artician skill which we have gathered from old excavations. The method of primitive healings was not concentrated on logic and Scientific data but on belief and crude methods of transference of evil spirits and using certain methods like herbs or animal extracts which was the monopoly of certain group of people. It may be said that it is a mere method of exploitation than a process of real healing and occasionally it occurred some natural processes of healing, which was claimed as their credit or hereditary monopoly.

Study of Folk medicine reveals many curious beliefs and creeds, a very important part of medical history. The use of remedies was not

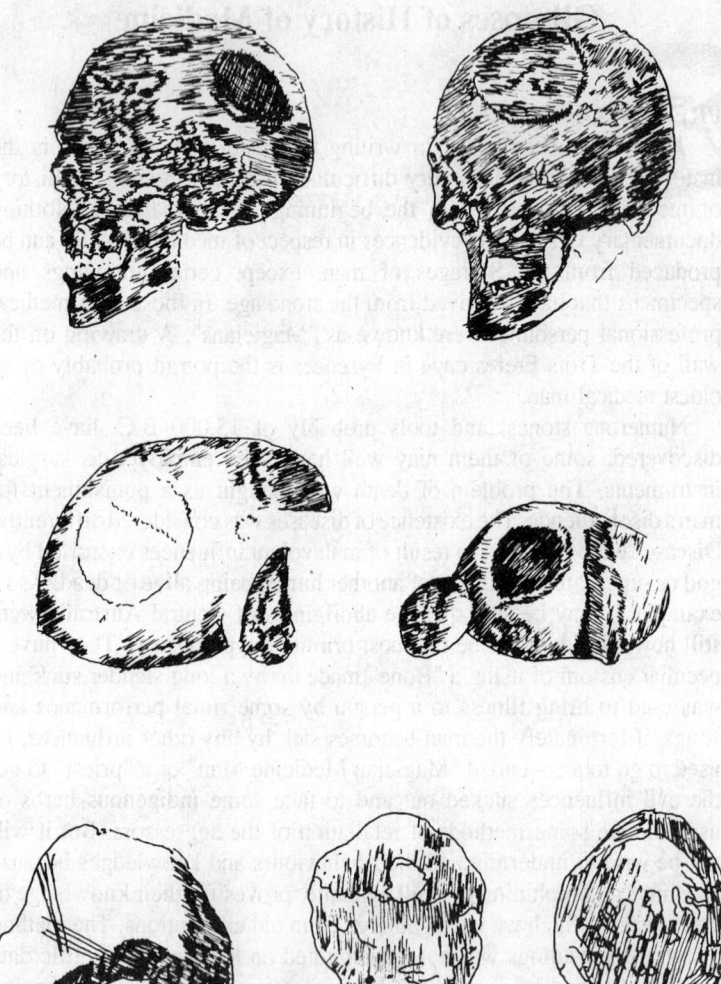

Fig. 1   Skull of early Bronze age with large trephined opening found in crichel down, Dorset in 1938. Fig. on Right shows excised bone replaced.
Fig. 1.a   Experiment to illustrate trephining by means of a flint scaper, showing two stages of the operation.
Fig. 1.b   Cranial amulets from dolmens in France. (L) an irregular fragment with margin of trephined hole in the centre of the lower margin (1.5 CM natural size). The perforated for use as "Charm".

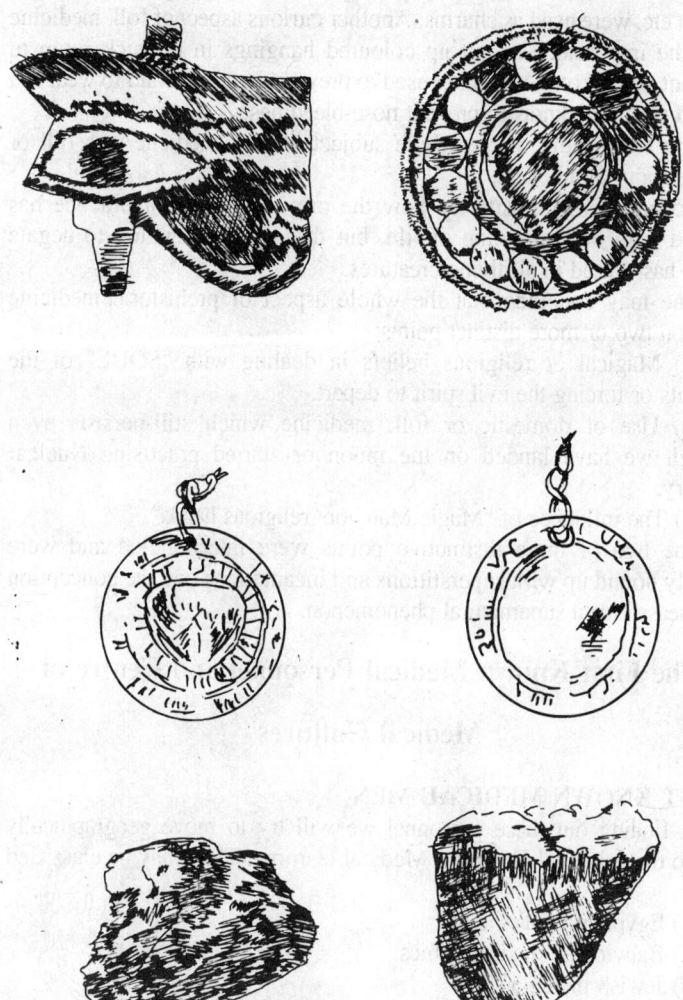

CHARMS AMULETS TALISMAN

Fig. 2   (L) Ancient Egyptian enamel charm representing the eye of Hous.
(R) Amulets inscribed "Richardson's Magneto-Galvanic Battery sold as cure for Rheumatism.

Fig. 2.a The Leepenny or Talisman.

Fig. 2.b (L) Wart-like stone from ottery St. Mary, Devon 1910 used for curing warts.
(R). Stone resembling a tooth, used to cure toothache.

only internal but used to be carried as charms and talismans, as a part of treatment. The skin of a snake, the patella of a sheep, the nail of a coffin etc. were used as charms. Another curious aspect of folk medicine was the importance to put up coloured hangings in the sick room to prevent small-pox, red flannel used to prevent sorethroat and to wear red thread with nine knots to prevent nose-bleedings.

The basic thing of the whole subject of folk medicne was full of superstitions and beliefs.

No one knows positively how the origin of Medical practice has started with the beginning of life, but the idea of negation to negate death has started in all living creatures.

One may conclude that the whole aspect of prehistoric medicine rests on two or more distinct points:

(1) Magical or religious beliefs in dealing with "SOUL" of the patients or forcing the evil spirit to depart.

(2) Use of domestic or folk medicine which still-persists even though we have landed on the moon or started practising Nuclear surgery.

(3) The influence of "Magic Man" or "religious heads".

The two or three distinctive points were intermingled and were closely bound up with superstitions and incantations and the conception of disease was a supernatural phenomenon.

The First Known Medical Personnel and Centre of Medical Cultures

FIRST KNOWN MEDICAL MEN

In finding out these personnel we will try to move geographically and to the principal Centre of Medical learning. They may be classified as :

(1) Egyptian medicine.
(2) Babylonian medical ethics.
(3) Jewish medicine.
(4) India's ancient medicine.
(5) Chinese medicine.
(6) Greece and Roman medicine.

EGYPTIAN MEDICINE

Between the northern boundary of Arabian desert and the mountains of Asia Minor there was a fertile crescent of land. There developed a great civilization known at first as "SUMERIAN" and latter as the kingdoms of "SUMER" and "AKKAD". These civilisations were sensible organisations of society consisting of learned people, military and industrial classes of personnel.

Our main sources of Egyptian medicine are the "MEDICAL PAPYRI", "CLAY TABLET" and exacavated material like small knives. Archcological excavations, old manuscripts, wall writings, old paintings and engravings in the doors of tombs of the burial grounds have revealed many lights. The seal of a Sumerian physician of 3000 B.C. is still kept in the Welcome Museum. Similarly there is a seal of a Babylonian medical man of 2300 B.C.

The earliest known picture or excavated skeleton of Surgical operation during the regime of 5th dynasty (2750-2625 B.C.) gave evidence of well-splinted fractures and their knowledges.

The medicine chest box of an Egyptian queen of 11th dynasty containing vases, spoons, dried drugs and roots is an important finding in support of their medical thoughts. But whatever may be the origin of medical practice it was based on magical and religious beliefs connected with the "SOUL" of the patients or in persuading or forcing the evil spirit which has entered the body of the patients.

What-so-ever the surgical methods or trephining were used, the basic idea was to drive out the evil spirit bound up by superstitions, incantations and this conception of supernatural phenomenon persisted for long long years. The superstitions were so great that they used to take a hair of the dog that had bitten.

Egyptian and Sumerians were staying side by side with the Palestines as an intervening country. They were culturally and commercially interlinked with each other and so also their medical beliefs and traditions.

Hammurabi (1848-105 B.C.), one of the earliest king of Babylon, drew up a code of Medical Ethics, which is still preserved and which seems to be the oldest Medical ethics.

In the ethics it was stated that if a doctor shall treat a gentleman and open an abscess with knife and may preserve the eye of the patient the doctor will get ten silver shekels and in the case of a slave the master will have to pay two silver shekels. On the reverse, if the doctor kills the patients or destroys the eyes his hands may be taken off in the case of a gentleman and in case of a slave the doctor will have to replace the slave. Nucleus of everything in the medical thoughts was relating to some sorts of God or supernatural power and their influences.

THOTH, the ibis headed GOD of wisdom, was said to be the author of Medical treatise, the lion headed SEKHMET was the deity of childbirth. HORUS was the GOD of Health. HORUS lost one of his eyes in a fight with SET, the demon of evil. Ultimately the eye was restored by miraculous means. The eye of Horus formed the design of a charm; the design of the eye is said to be the origin of receipe (Rx). Originally an elaborate design, of the eye of Horus passed through various phases until it resembled like the capital (R) and it was placed on all objects associated with danger such as ships, chariots and prescriptions. The names of the numerous GODs were synthatized to form the famous GOD of medicine IMHOTEP.

But it will be futile attempt for us to point out, who was really the first Medical man. It may be SEKHET or IMHOTEP.

To many of us instead of IMHOTEP or AESCULAPIUS as GOD of healing HIPPOCRATES is regarded as really the father of medicine. No history of medicine shall be complete unless the strange customs of preserving the human body after death by injecting Cedar Wood oil, immersing in salt water and taking out the brain matter through nostril, putting cassia and other spices or drugs or preservatives in emptied abdominal cavity are studied. These cadavers were bandaged and soaked in heated resin. These were called as MUMMIES and were kept in temples or tombs with certain writings which had helped us to know something of the past creeds, customs and superstitions. This method of preservation has not helped much to gain knowledge of Anatomy and Pathology or cause of diseases, as the people were not inclined to know Post-mortems as they were made for the idea of preservations only.

During the search for knowledge of medicine of old times, one has to refer to the BIBLE. In the BIBLE there is an absence of medicine or surgery but there are lots of information regarding personal and social Hygiene. Physical purity was considered as a complementary to moral purity and cleanliness was literally next to godliness. Individuals were considered only a part of a community. It tries to increase the social conscience.

No account of the first known medical man or medical practice will be completed until and unless reference of the East is made, specially that of INDIA (HINDUS) and CHINA and Egyptians. The earliest Sanskrit documents the RIGVEDA (about 1500 B.C.) indicates the treatment of diseases mainly by spells and incantations.

Latter a series of works called AYUR-VEDA (about 700 B.C.) contains much medical information. CHARAKA and SUSRUTA were among the contributors. But the first original book was made before those great Hindu Physicians. CHARAK lived in the beginning of Christian era and SUSRUTA lived about fifth century A.D. Susruta wrote about Malaria caused by mosquitoes, Plague followed when many dead rats were seen and Phthisis showed by Haemoptysis, fever and

FIRST KNOWN MEDICAL MAN
Fig. 3 Statuette of Imhotep physician and vizier to king Zoser about 2980 B.C.

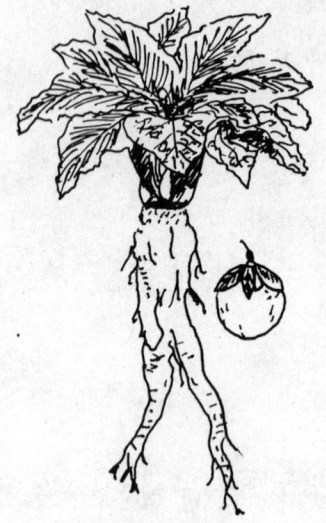 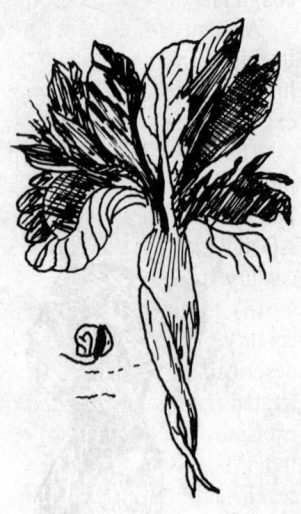

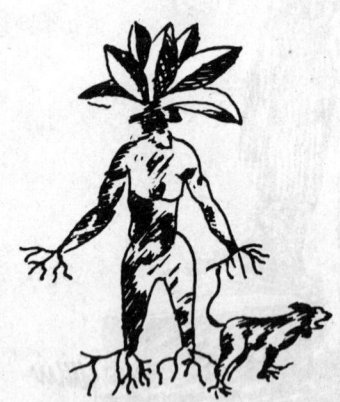 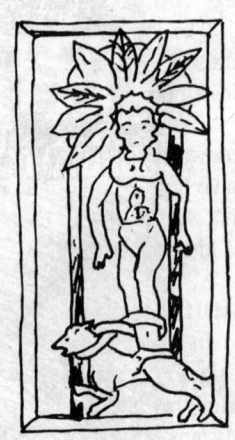

Fig. 4 Mandragora, or Mandrake, as represented in early herbals, showing the fancied resemblance of the plant to the human figure.

Fig. 4.b (L) Mandragora, with the dog used in gathering the root (from an early edition of the Herbal of Apuleius). (R) A more fanciful version of the mandragora legend by an Anglo-Saxon artist of the thirteenth century.

cough and also gave description of small pox.

Ancient Hindus were extremely good in Surgery. In an Indian rock inscription, king Asoka (226 B.C.) records the erection of Hospitals by him. India and Ceylon were one country. Cingalese records indicate the existence of Hospitals in Ceylon in 437 and 137 B.C.

The three leading text books of Hindu medicine which were mainly predominated by the Brahmin priests and scholars are the (i) Charaka Samhita, a compendium made by CHARAK from an earlier works of AGNIVERA, based upon the lectures of his master ATREYA (6th century B.C.)

(ii) the SUSRUTA (5th century A.D.), (iii) VAGBHATA (7th century A.D.). Of these the most remarkable is Susruta. SUSRUTA described more than a HUNDRED SURGICAL instruments. Hindus treated fractures with bamboo splints and performed caesarean Section, excision of tumours, lithotomy and rhinoplasty which originated in India. Hindu medicine was very rich in drugs. SUSRUTA mentioned seven hundred and sixty medicinal plants, ointments, baths, sneezing powders and inhalations which were used as external applications. Hindus may be called as pioneers of modern Plastic Surgery.

Diabetes Mellitus was recognised as "MADHU MEHA" and the symptoms of thirst, foul breath and general weakness were noted. Evidence of inoculation against small pox has been found in Sanskrit text "SACTEYA" attributed to Dhanwantari.

The Hindu system of Respiratory exercises or gymnastic is highly praised till to-day. In Marcopolo's travel experience there is a description of a kind of Mosquito netting used on the coromandal coast.

The Soporitic effects of Hyoscyamus and Cannabis Indica were known to the Hindu Surgeons as Surgical Anesthesia. The Hindus may have borrowed something from the Greek. Some writers even maintain that Aristotle who lived at the last part of real Hindu culture got some of his ideas from the east.

MOHAMMEDAN AND JEWISH PERIOD

In Mohammedan Culture and religion the sacred and Holy word "Islam" means resigned unconditional submission to the will of Almighty GOD. The popularity of names Iskandar, Ibrahim, Ismail, Miriam showed the evidence of close contact of Mohammedans with Greek and Jewish culture.

As such in the field of medicine the principle of practice Greek influences were predominated yet the SARACENS themselves were the originator not only of Algebra, chemistry and geology but many improvements and refinements of civilization both in personal hygienic customs and public measures.

The true starting point of Mohammedan medicine was made by eastablishing the famous school "GONDISAPOR".

The greatest physicians RHAZES, HALY ABBAS and IBN SINA (Avicenna).

HALY BEN ABBAS: A persian who died in 994 was the author of the ALMAL KI (Royal book) which was a great treatise and guide on medicine for a hundred years which was later on superseded by the CANON of Avicenna. It was translated into Latin at about 1070-80, it contains a description of small pox and "Persian fire (malignant anthrax).

IBN SINA (980-1037) was called as the "Prince of Physician".

His wonderful description of the origin of mountains entitled him to be called as father of Geology and it is interesting to note that two physicians widely separated in space and time—Avicenna and Fracastorius are the only writers who contributed anything of value to the science.

CANON, a treatise was a huge store house of learning, in which the author attempted to codify the whole medical knowledge of his time.

He was said to have been the first to describe the preparation and properties of sulphuric acid and alcohol. He gave a good description of Gunea-worm.

RHAZES (860-932) was a great clinician. His description of small pox, measles was the first authentic accounts in literature. He had a great encyclopedia of medicine known as EL HAW.

USEI BIA (120-69) of Damascus, the first medical historian who wrote a series of biographies of ancient physicians ISSAC JUDAEUS— a Jewish physician. His other name was Issac Israeli of Kaironan. He wrote a book on uroscopy and a most popular book on Dietetics.

IBN AL HAITHAM or known as Alhazan of Bassora whose Theasurus of OPTICS contains the first note of occular refraction and of the fact that a segment of a glass ball will magnify objects.

ALBUCASIS (1013) born in the Andalusian a town zahra near Cordva was the author of the great Medio-Chirrgical treatise called ALTASRIF. It contained illustrations of surgical and dental instruments and was the leading text book of surgery. It consisted of three volumes: The first one deals with the use of actual CAUTERY, a special feature of the Arabian Surgery and gave descriptions and figures of peculiar instruments, the second one contained full description of "Lithotomy", "Lithotrily", "Amputation for gangrene" and different treatment of wounds, the third volume deals with "Fractures and Dislocations including fractures of Pelvis and mention of paralysis in fracture of the spine.

He first wrote on the treatment of deformities of the mouth and dental arches and mentioned the obstetric posture which is now known, as "WALCHER POSTURE".

AVENZOAR: He was the greatest of the Mohammedan physicians of the western caliphate. He died in the year 1162. His elaborate description of ITCH-MITE had given him possibly the first Parasitologist after Alexander of Tralles. He gave description of paralysis and inflammation of the middle ear and recommended goats milk in Phthisis. He had the courage to go against the then galenism.

AVERROES (1126-1198): He was a spanish Moslem. He was more noted as a philosopher and as a free thinker than a physician. His KITAB-AL-KULLYAT was an attempt to find a system of medicine upon the customary neo-Platonic modification of Aristotle's Philosophy.

ABU MANSUR: He was a man of repute. His book on materia medica was the important persian work on Pharmacology. It contained description of 585 drugs of which 466 were vegetables, 75 minerals and 44 animals origin. The Arabic Writings on TOXICOLOGY upto the end of 12th century was considered as an exhaustive and authenticated one.

The Arabians were able chemists and good Pharmacologists also. Their description of materia medica and preparation of drugs become standard authority throughout the middle ages.

MEDICAL CULTURE OF MOHAMMEDANS

The Arabians derived their knowledge of Greek medicine from Nestorians monks and many practical details from the Jews and their astrological conception from the Egyptians and from east. The essential features of Arabian physicians training was that most had extensive knowledge of Mohammedan theology, Law, Philosophy, astronomy, astrology, other parts of Arts, science and medicine. They must have to be acquainted with the Galenical system of medicine. Their diagnosis of internal diseases were founded upon from Six canons: (1) the patient's action, (2) his or her excreta, (3) the nature of the pain, (4) its site, (5) swelling, (6) effluvia of the body; further information were cited from the feel of the hand, yellowness of the eye and bending of the back.

The symptoms of yellow bile reflects a shallow complexion, dryness of the throat, a bitter taste, loss of appetite, rapid pulse and those of black bile was false appetite and great mental disquiet and *cark* and care terminating in melancholia.

They abstained from dissecting out of religious conviction, left operative surgery and venesection to the wandering specialists and obstetric cases to the midwives.

The best and the largest of the Mohammedan Hospitals were at Damascus (1160) and at Cairo (1276).

The AL-MANSUR Hospital at Cairo (1283) was large enough with beautifully decorated. It employed male and female nurses. Medical teachings were probably given at Bagdad, Damascus and Cairo. The principle courses were clinical medicine, pharmacology and therapeutics. Anatomy and Surgery were neglected, chemistry was given special importance.

Arabian medicine was, infact, the parent of Alchemy, the founder of which was JABU or GEBER (702-765), the discoverer of Nitric acid, regia and the discoverer of distillation, filtration, sublimation, water baths.

With the faded glory of the Greece and Rome, Medicine passed into the hands of two classes: (i) Arabian Scholars, (ii) Christian Church.

In the early part of the medical science Christian Churches were very conservative and it could not be denied that they contributed almost nothing towards the progress of science, but really retarded the progress of medical science.

The Christian view of disease was a retrograde vice.

Human body was considered sacred and its dissection was prohibited; a veto was imposed by the church and also by the Mohammedans.

It was denied that diseases had natural origin. Many diseases were considered as punishments for sin.

Though the Arabians tried their best to construct their medicine in a logical and regular manner without much knowledge of anatomy and physiology.

Some of the details of Arabian medicine have been discussed in the previous chapter, the christian era slightly improved with establishing the SCHOOL OF SALERNO and full domination of Patron Saints in medicine came in question.

People were made to believe on Partian saints who were thought to occupy various parts of human body; SAINT BLAISE dominated the throat, SAINT BERNARDINE the lung, SAINT APOLLONIA the teeth, SAINT LAWRENCE the back, SAINT ERASMUS the abdomen.

SCHOOL OF SALERO: Salero was a charming town at seaside approximately 35 miles from Naples. It was the seat of first organised medical school.

It is said, the school was founded by four masters: Elinus the Jew,

Pontus the Greek, Adale the Arbian and Salermus the Latin.

Though there was no valuable discovery but the epoch of the Renaissance which started later on was established at Salerno.

There were some renowned persons like GARIOPONTUS (1050). BARTHOLOMEUS ANGLICUS compiled some important medical books like "Passionaries Practice".

It is a great matter of interesting that Ladies who had medical training from Salerno like TROTULA, ABELLA, REBECCA, CONSTANZA and other, whose names were found in the history. Trotula also wrote a book on obstetrics (1050 A.D.).

Medical teaching was not haphazard at Salerno. In this early twelfth century medical practice was brought under official jurisdiction by king. Roger II of Sicily and later on by Emperor Frederick II.

It was decided that no one could practise medicine until and unless he had been examined and approved by the Masters of Salerno. This legislation was made to avoid danger from the inexperience of the physician. The course was of five years and minimum age for admission was twenty one years after passing the examination; the candidates had to take an oath "To uphold the School", "to attend to the poor without any charges", "to administer no noxious drug", "to teach nothing false", "Not to keep an apothecary's shop". He/She was awarded a Ring, a laurel wreath, a book and the kiss of peace.

Thus the medicine in the 11th and 12th century was lifted to a much higher level by the School of Salerno. This little place was a seaside town of Salerno near Naples; was known to the Romans as an ideal Health resort. It is said that the school of Salerno was founded by the four masters: a greek, a Latin, a Jew and a Saracen. The influence of Greek was prominent.

When the Moslem power (827-884) had their rule over Sicily and Southern part of Italy; Arabic medical doctrine infused with the Western European culture until its existence.

The advent of Constantinus Africanus is the period of greatest literary activity of the school Salerno.

The main source of Anatomical knowledge was Constantine's translation of Almaleki (Royal book) written by HALY BEN ABBAS, a persian magnus, who was the author that treatise on matters medical. Constantinus Africanus translated it into Latin (1070-80) and later another translation was made by Stephen of Antioch.

12 and 13th Century (Mediaeval Period): Really the medical period in Europe started from 476 to 1453 B.C. but in the Indian continent it started from the beginning of the Mohammedan rule upto the end of Moghal period.

The history of medicine in mediaeval period of Europe is regarded as an age of decadence and of stagnation and the very name mediaeval implies the negation at progress and suggests backwardness, superstition and sloth.

The then conception of disease was archaic, diagnosis and prognosis were based on the state of stars and inspection of urine, treatment consisted of blood letting and using some herbs whose actions were not well defined. But in this long period of the centuries some light was seen with full faiths of Galenic misconceptions Schools of medicine were opened.

The Medical school of MONTPELLIER was opened possibly in 12th century. Montpellier was a health resort like Salerno.

People could easily go to Montpellier from Spain and Italy.

It was renowned during the 13th and 14th century. Many famous people were attached with this. After the rise of medical school at Padua its fame gradually came but it continued its celebration upto 1890.

ARNOLD of VILLANOVA spent most of his life at Montpillier. In the 16th century his book known as "BREVIARIUM PRACTICE" was well circulated. He was both a surgeon and physician. His advice as a surgeon was "to postpone opening an abscess is dangerous" "The bite of mad dog should be enlarged and encouraged to bleed".

He found out that the virtues of herbs could be extracted by alcohol Martpeller attracted many English and French people.

Among them was BERNARD DE GORDOM who contributed in the field of medicine. In his writings "LILIUM MEDICINAE" he gave description of a "TRUSS" and the first mention of SPECTACLES.

In between Rome and Padua there was a famous city known as BOLOGNA. In Bologna there was a famous school of law, a school of Anatomy and Surgery was established later on.

The university of Paris and Padua took leading places in the history of medicine.

GUIDO LANFRANCHI (D 1315): A distinguished surgeon who fled from Italy to France and settled in Paris. He was a reputed surgeon and teacher. In his book CHIRURGIA MAGNA he mentioned the importance of careful suture of the ends of the divided nerve.

In the meantime university of PADUA a university which played a great part in the renaissance of medical learning came up.

Apart from medical learning two great Scholars, one of them an English Franciscan and another a German Dominion exercised much influence upon the intellectual life of the time.

FRANCISCAN ROGER BACON (1214-1294) was a great scholar with idea far ahead of his time and it might be out of place as mediaeval figure.

His work was appreciated many years after his death.

He incurred displeasure of the church and was imprisoned for fourteen years. Many of his writings are still unpublished. His first work "OPUSMAJUS" was printed in 1733.

He was not a physician but a physicist, mathematician and logical philosopher.

He had been credited rightly or wrongly with the invention of telescope, the microscope, the diving bell, spectacles and foretelling mechanical transport.

He was forerunner of inductive and experimental science.

Medicine he regarded as a means of prolonging of life through alchemy (Chemistry). He approved of astrology and other modes of superstition on account of their psycho-therapeutic effect. His principal contributions to medical literature are his astrological tracts on critical days.

Associated with Roger Bacon there was in Paris ALBERT VON BOLSTAOT, a Dominiean monk, was a close follower and interpreter of Aristotle.

He was not only a philosopher or a theologist but was an authority on the healing virtues of plant and wrote a book (DE VEGETABILIBUS).

Restoration of Anatomy Teacher

Before the advent of vesalius the great painter of the renaissance period were making dissections in the hospitals at Florence (Santo Spirite). Milan and Rome, but apart from artists like Leonard—Da-Vinci whose paintings really advanced Anatomy without didactic intention, dissection was mainly a show and ornamental feature of the mediaeval period.

Pope Boniface VIII put up a mandate for not destroying dead crusaders by boiling the dead bodies and returning the bones to their relatives. It helped to dissect the dead bodies which was an indirect help.

The value of anatomy though gained recognition in the later part of middle but the teaching was started more on theoretical basis and ten heads of the state or religion felt the need of dissecting human body and this pope was one of them. For sudicial reasons Post-mortem examination was practised and executed criminals were publicly dissected. This dissection was generally carried by the menials and the Professor used to pointout from a far distant height. It was not a systematic dissection.

The first attempt to remedy this condition of affairs and to introduce the systematic teaching was made by MONDINO DE LUZZI or Mudinus (1275-1326). Under his guidance Anatomy became recognised as the essential part in Medical curriculum. His book "ANOTHOMIA" written in 1316 is the first practical Manual in Anatomy. Many of his anatomical terms were Arabic—(Abdominal—Wall—Minach, Peritoneum—Siphac, Omentum—Zirbus). There were errors made by Yalen and the descriptions were superficials.

Alongwith this a student of Mundinus—GUY DE CHAULIAC, the son of French peasant studied medicine and theology at Montpellier and Bologna and became the physician to Pope at Avigon clement VI and his two successors. He was a good surgeon and insisted that knowledge and practice of Surgery stand on good knowledge of Anatomy.

No account of Mediaeval medicine will be completed until a short description of the wide spread epidemic of Plague (BLACK DEATH) which devasted the world in the fourteenth century is given. It caused the death of the quarter of the population. Half of the London population died. Dead bodies were thrown in the North sea and the mediterranian and spread the infection in the central Asia to Europe.

The history of the mediaeval period will not be completed if certain names are not recorded, like ROGER (Reggiero Frugardi) of Palermo, RCNALD (Ranaldo Capelluti) of Parma, SALICETO (1210-1277), HENI HENRI De-MONDEVILL (1260-1320), Peter D' ARGELTA (? 1423), a Professor of Bolagna JOHN OF ARDERNE (1306-90), GUV-de CHAULIAC (1300-68), ROGER II, FREDERICK II.

ROGER: They were writers of independent thoughts and were not influence of Coustantinus Africanus, Rogers work became a standard book at Salerno. He knew cancer and possibly syphilis, a case of Hernia of lungs, Iodine (spange and sea wood) for goitre, mercusial ointment for chronic and dermal affections use of styptics, suture and ligature in Haemorrhage, healing wounds by second intention. SALICETO: He was the ablest Italian surgeon of 13th century and was a professor at Bolagna.

He wrote a book on Internal Medicine and surgery also. He did not separate the surgical diagnosis from internal medicine. One of his treatise was the first known treatise in regional or surgical Anatomy. He showed how to suture a divided nerve and to diagnosis bleeding from an artery by the spurt of blood and specific contralateral paralysis as a sequel of head injuries.

HERI de MONDEVILLE (1260-1320) was a surgeon of original thinking. The surgical treatise of Mandiville of 1306 was well recognised which continued upto 1893 in different languages. He was a surgeon of depending on Natural healing process and advised that the wound should be washed to keep it clean.

Another surgeon known as PIETRO-D-A-RGELATA who died in 1423 who was Professor at Bologna. He also wrote a CIRURGIA which was printed in Venice in 1480.

He showed technique of embaling the corpse of Allexondar V. He was very skilled in dentistry and triphining the skull and incising the line a able in postmortem cearian section and was a skilled operator for Hearnia, stone and fistula-in-Ano. The fistula Ano operation was improved and attended with a high degree of perfection in the hands of JOHN OF ARDERNA. JOHN was also a skilled surgeon and also devised many new surgical instruments. He employed irrigation in a renal and intestinale Colic, systitis and gonorrhoea.

During Mediaeval period along with the surgery, there were efforts to improve the Status of the Human Anatomy. Initially desction is perfomr but later on it was prescribed by how to have dissections once or twice a year. The only Text books of Anatomy were Anatomia of Richard of Wen dover and Anatomia Vivorum.

GUYDE CHAULIAC (1300-68): He was a prominent product of mont pallir and was a good surgeon. During this period the medicine in Britane was entirely in the hands of a corporation of magician and those who had assumed Iatro Mentic functions.

In the Russia the medicine was originaly in the hands of VOLKHAVA OR WALFAMAN who used medicinal herbs and used charms and spells.

Throughout this there were some vague attempts to formulate the principle of medical Jurisprudence.

In the year 1140. Roger II of Sicily issued am edict forbidding anyone to practise medicine without proper examination, under pain of imprisonment and the sale of his belongings at auction. This important law was followed by an ordinance of larger scope issued by Roger's grandson, the generous and liberal-mined Hohenstauffen Emperor, Frederick II in 1242.

Another important fact, thrown into relief by the 15th century pictures, is that the use of spectacles had by this time become quite common. They were introduced about 1270-80 by the glass-workers of Venice.

One of the earliest teachers of medicine at Bologna were two surgeons father and son Theodric (1205-98) was the illustrious son of the surgepon's father. He combined theology with medicine which was the fashion of the Mediaeval period become the Bishop of cr. cerveia. He used to practise in surgery and wrote certain notable commands like the formation pus in wounds is unnecessary and undesirable also. He used to an anaesthetic sponge impregnated with a herbal known as Mandragra and Opium. This Mandragra. On Mandrake is one of the most ancient herbal remedies. This plant is common in the Mediterranean area and has a long top roof often befed and bears to some resemblance to the human figure. The plant has two arities (male & female) which may be distingused easily.

CHINESE: History of Chinese Medicine is not only noteworthy but is well—worthy of investigation study. SHEN NUNG, a Chinese emperor who lived about 3000 B.C. is called as a father of medicine. He made experiment upon himself and wrote book PEN TSOAS (Chinese Materia Medica). It contains description of thousand drugs. Vegetable substances like opium, Rhubarb, Aconite, Croton; inorganic substances like iron, arsenic, Sulphur, were mentioned. Ephedrine an alkalied were isolated from a Chinese herb MAHUANG. Another emperor HWANGT (2650) is said to be the author of another book known as NEICHING, the book of medicine. It is said that before harvey Chinese discovered the circulation of blood from the heart. Their broad principles were based on two opposing principles YANG and YIN like life and death, male and female, sun and moon, ebb and flow and five elements: earth, fire, water, wood, metal. This figure of five were applied to the organs of body (heart, liver, spleen, lung, kidney) and to various other objects like colour, climate and heavenly bodies. Health was considered as a harmonius balance.

Massages and Acupuncture were practised from very ancient times. Inoculation against small pox was practised in China. Dead crust from small pox were used as snuff in the nose. Two famous medical personalities are worthy to name. CHANG CHUNG KING (195 A.D.) is called as Chinese Hippocratic, because of his observatory facts (Treatment of fever). HUATU (115-205 A.D.) was a famous surgeon of China. He used anaesthesia before operating upon patients (? CANNABIS INDICA) as anacthesia. He has described two hundred varieties of pulse and diseases may be diagnosed by the pulse. a system of practice by old Hindu practitioners known as Aurved.

The first Chinese to study medicine abroad was WONG FOON, who graduated in Edinberg in 1885 and practised at Canton. His pioneer work was the foundation of Hospitals and medical School.

JAPAN: Orginaly medicine was under the influence of China but later on influence of Germany become prominent and German was adopted as the language of scientific periodicals.

Japan made noteworthly contributions to the progress in bacteriology. Among them who led the way were such men like KITASATD (1852-1931).

Who worked under Kock for six years and discovered the bacillus of Plague in 1894.

HINDEYO NOGUCHI (1876-1928)

He was research fellow an yellow fever, but died on yellow fever.

Though empiricism and superstition were dominating, ancient Greece was forerunner in the branch of medicine like other branches of History, philosophy, mathematics, astronomy, sculpture. Babylon, Egypt, Persia. India transmitted many thoughts to Greece.

Incubation as method of cure were practised favourable by diet, bathing, exercise, physical therapy.

Among the Greek philosopher PYTHAGORAS (580-489 B.C.) and his school which he founded exercised a profoud influence upon medicine. They taught men to inquire into causes for the sake of knowledge. ALCMAEON of Croton a student of Pythagoras dissected on annual. The optic nerve, distinguished between veins and arteries, brain the seat of sense and intellect.

EMPEDOCIES (504-443): He lived in Agrigentem in Sicily was another follower of Pythagoras school. He regarded the universe and everything in it is composed of four elements: Fire, Air, Earth, Water are considered. Health is the equipoise and disease is the preponderance of Heat, Cold, Moisture, Dryness, Acidity, Sweatness. Presence of optic nerve, head of the foetus first to develope, brain the seat of higher activity and the origin of nerve was thought by Empedodes.

HIPPOCRATES was born in 460 B.C. in the island of Cos close to Asia Minor.

The collections of Hippocratic (CORPU HIPPOCRATICUM) have been translated in many languages and in studying the works no one can fail remark his high standard of ethical conduct, his insistence of prognosis, his accuracy of observations and his clarity of recording cases. He was the first man to separate Medicine from Philosophy and set up a high standard of ethics who wished to follow the ART of medicine.

Hipporcates knew little of Anatomy and Physiology. He had not the Clinical thermometer nor stethoscope, yet he practised AUSCULTATION by placing ear to the chest and able to describe the friction sound of the pleurisy as creaking of leather.

He openly denied the theory that diseases have some divine or sacred relationship. He tried to find out the real causes of Epilepsy or fever. The logical writings of the different observatory facts are seen in the different aphorisms.

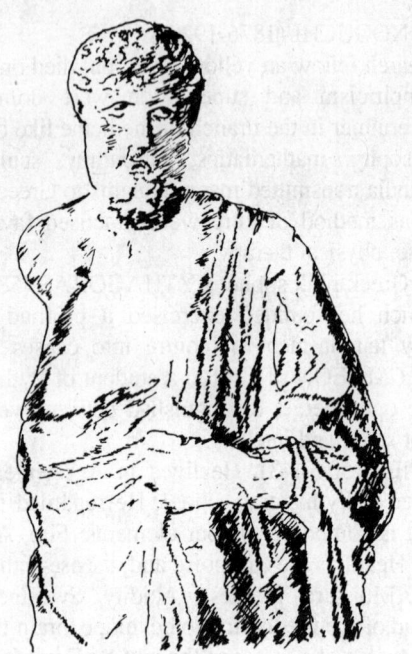

THE FATHER OF MEDICINE

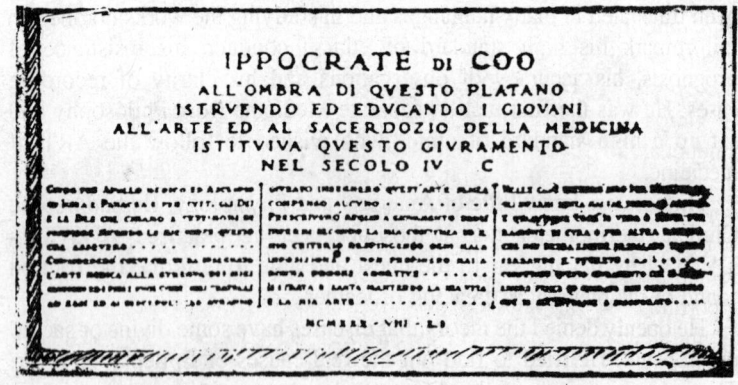

Fig. 5   Upper-Statue found on the island COS, believed to be that of HIPPOCRATES.
Italian inscription at the base of the "The tree of Hippocrates in Cos.

Aphorisms and Oath of Hippocratic

The Oath is worth quoting in its entirety in one of the numerous English renderings:

"I swear by Apollo the Physician, by Aesculapius, by Hygeia, by Panacea, and by all the gods and goddesses, making them my witnesses, that I will carry out according to my ability and judgment, this oath and this indenture. To hold my teacher in this art equal to my own parents; to make him partner in my livelihood; when he is in need of money to share mine with him; to consider his family as my own brothers, and to teach them this art, if they want to learn it, without fee or indenture; to impart precept, oral instruction, and all other instruction to my own sons, the sons of my teacher, and to pupils who have taken the physicians' Oath, but to nobody else. I will use treatment to help the sick according to my ability and judgment, but never with a view to injuring and wrong-doing. Neither will I administer a poision to anybody when asked to do so, nor will I suggest such a course. Similarly I will not give to a woman a pessary to cause abortion. But I will keep pure and holy both my life and my art. I will not use the knife, not even verily, on sufferers from stone, but I will give place to such as are craftsmen therein. Into whatsoever houses I enter, I will enter to help the sick, and I will abstain from all intentional wrongdoing and harm, especially from abusing the bodies of man or woman, bond or free. And whatsoever I shall see or hear in the course of my profession, as well as outside my profession in my intercourse with men, if it be what should not be published abroad. I will never divulge, holding such things to be holy secrets. Now if I carry out this oath, and break it not may I gain for ever reputation among all men for my life and for my art; but if I transgress it and forswear myself, may the opposite befall me".

Various embellishments of the oath and hints on professional conduct are to be found in other Hippocratic writings. The book entitled precepts, generally believed to be of later date than Hippocrates, but the work of one of his school, gives the following advice: "I urge you not to be too grasping, but to consider carefully your patient's means. Sometimes give your services for nothing.... and if there be an opportunity of serving one who is a stranger in financial straits, of serving one who is a stranger in financial straits, give full assistance to all such. For where there is the love of man, there is also of the art". (Prec.vi.)

Hippocrates did not confine his practice to medicine. He was a good surgeon. He drained pus, set fractures, and reduced dislocations (using a special bench or table), and even trephined the skull, as he clearly describes in the work on wounds in the Head. His use of tar for wounds is surprising forerunner of the antiseptic method. Even more remarkable is the advice which he gives in his short note-book entitled, in the Surgery.

The "Aphorisms"

No account of Hippocrates is complete without some reference to his famous Aphorisms. The first of these is almost hackneyed. "Life is short, and the Art long; opportunity fleeting; experiment dangerous, and judgment difficult," he writes, and he goes on to advise the doctor to be prepared to do the right thing at the right time, in which "patient, attendants, and external circumstances must co-operate."

A few of the other aphorisms may be quoted, as they illustrate so well the teaching of the great master:

I. 6. For extreme diseases extreme strictness of treatment is most efficacious.

I. 13. Old men endure fasting most easily, the man of middle age, youths very badly, and worst of all children, especially those of a liveliness greater than the ordinary.

I. 20. Do not disturb a patient either during or just after a crisis, and try no experiments, neither with purges nor with other irritants, but leave him alone.

II. 2. When sleep puts an end to delirium it is a good sign.

II. 16. When on starvation diet a patient should not be fatigued.

II. 33. In every disease it is a good sign when the patient's intellect is sound and he enjoys his food; the opposite is a bad sign.

II. 39. Old men generally have less illness than young men, but such complaints as become chronic in old men generally last until death.

III. 16. The diseases which generally arise in rainy weather are protracted fevers, fluxes of the bowels, mortifications, epilepsy, apoplexy, eye diseases of the joints, strangury and dysentery.

III. 19. All diseases occur at all seasons, but some diseases are more apt to occur and to be aggravated at certain seasons.

III. 23. In winter occur pleurisy, pneumonia, colds, sore throat, headache, dizziness, apoplexy.

II. 24. In the different ages the following complaints occur : to little children and babies aphthae, vomitting, coughs, sleeplessness, terrors, watery discharges from the ears.

III. 31. Old men suffer from difficulty in breathing, catarrh accompanied by coughing difficult, micturition pains at the joints, dizziness, apoplexy, pruritus, watery discharges from the bowels, ears and nostrils, dullness of sight, hardness of hearing.

V. 6. Those who are attacked by tetanus either die in four days, or, if they survive these, recover.

V. 9. Consumption occurs chiefly between the ages of eighteen and thirty-five.

V. 14. If diarrhoea attacks a consumptive patient it is a fatal symptom.

VI. 38. It is better to give no treatment in cases of hidden cancer: treatment causes speedy death, but to omit treatment is to prolong life.

VII. 34. When bubbles form in the urine it is a sign that the kidneys are affected and that the disease will be protracted.

VII. 72. Both sleep and sleeplessness, when beyond due measure, constitute disease.

VII. 87. Those diseases that medicines do not cure are cured by the knife. Those that the knife does not cure are cured by fire. Those that fire does not cure must be considered incurable.

Only a few of the aphorisms have been quoted, but they may suffice to illustrate the good sense and astute observation of the writer. Commentary is needless, to say that though hundreds of commentaries upon the aphorisms have been published, the originals deserve to be read and re-read by every practitioner of medicine and surgery. The work of Hippocrates is not a mere matter of historic interest. The idea of focusing full attention on the patient, rather than on scientific theories of disease or elaborate laboratory tests was revived by Sydenham and Boerhaave, and to-day it is again engaging the attention of some of the best minds in medicine. We cannot be too frequently or too forcefully reminded of the fact that "our natures are the physicians of our diseases." The physician and the specialist, whatever his field should study the entire patient and his environment, and should view disease with the eye of the naturalist. That is the message of Hippocrates, as fresh to-day as it was 2400 years ago.

From the study of the natural history of the disease he was able to forecast PROGNOSIS: The classical term "HIPPOCRATIC FACIES" came from the description of the face of an impending death.

It is described as : "Nose sharp, eyes hollow, temples shrunken, ears cold with their lobes turn outwart, the skin of the face parched and tense, the colour yellow or very dusky".

The position of the patient, nature of respiration, appearance of the Sputum, were stressed by him for prognosis.

But unfortunately he made little use of drug and depended on natural diet etc. (VIS MEDICATRIS NATURAE) for cure.

Aristotle and His Influence

Closely following Hippocrates in point of time was one who, though not himself a physician, exercised a profound influence upon the practice of medicine. ARISTOTLE (384-322 B. C.) was probably the greatest scientific genius the world has ever seen. He was not only a profound philosopher; his work as the first great biologist, was of inestimable value to medicine. His home was in Athens where he was a pupil of Plato, and later he was tutor to the son of Philip of Macedon, Alexander the Great.

He followed the Hippocrates and others in believing that human body possessed four fundamental qualities: the hot or cold, the dry and moist, and it composed of four "HUMOURS": the blood, phlegm, yellow bile and black bile.

Disturbance on the relative predominance of any of the humours constitute disease.

THEOPHRASTUS (370-287 B.C.): Aristotle was followed by Theophrastus. He was more a botanist than a Biologist. He laid the foundation of modern scientific world by writing a book "HISTORIA PLANTARUM".

He described not only the morphology and natural history of plants but also their THERAPEUTIC USE.

He showed the methods of collecting the extracts from the stem (collection of GUM) and described the process of germination of seeds and made a distinction between monocotyledons and dicotyledons.

DIOSCORIDES: A Greek surgeon to the army of Nero later on (60 A.D.) wrote a book on Materia Medica where he described the use of mineral remedies like salts of lead and copper.

THEOPHRASTUS: He was possibly the last scholars of the Greek medicine and the culture which shifted to the Romans.

ARISTOTLE (384-322 B. C.): He was born in Athens and was a student of Plato. He was not only a profound philosopher or a great biologist but an esteemed scholar in medicines.

Contributions of Aristotle

(1) Laid the foundations of comparative anatomy and embryology.

(2) Dissected on innumerable animals, specially on FISH and MOLLUSCUS.

(3) Gave a curious description of placental DOG FISH.

(4) Accurate description of the life of BEES and their ruler, the

queen.

(5) Gave a broad description of entire living world and their classification. In his conception of the ladder of the nature, indicated the primary belief of the theory of evolution.

Before rounding up the Hippocratic and his followers of Greek medicine, two persons of medical school of Alexandria are still remembered. They were born about 300 B. C.

ALEXANDRIA ROMAN medicine: (1) HEROPHILUS an anatomist. He is possibly the first person to practise public dissection of Human body. TORCULAR HEROPHILI, a venous sinus of the brain is named after him.

He was the first to name the Duodenum and to count the pulse.

(2) ERASISTRATUS founder of physiology. He distinguished the cerebrum and cerebellum and noted the difference between sensory and motor nerve. His beliefs were:

(a) Nerves are hollow tubes filled with fluid, air enter into the lung then to the heart and then changed into VITAL SPIRIT to be carried to the different parts of the body by arteries. Both of them practised human vivisection.

Among many of the Greek physicians who came to Rome ASCLEPIADES was called as Prince of Physician. He was born at Pursa in Bithynia on the south shore of Black sea in 124 B. C. on the south of Alexandria and ultimately settled in Rome.

He was the follower of Hippocrate but he denied to depend wholly on the nature for healing but in active to depend wholly on the nature for healing but in active measure by the physician. He originated the idea that diseases should be treated speedily, safely and agreeably. (CITO, TUTO, ET FUCUNDE).

To him Health was the balance between tension and relaxation.

This theory was known as "Methodism" was replaced in the later days by similar ideas by BROUSSAIS as theory of irritation and by BROWN as Brunonian theory of STHENIC and ASTHENIC States.

During this period a king Mithridates VI King of Pontus discovers certain antidotes to venomous reptile and poisonous substance. The drugs known as MITHRIDATICUM and THERIAC. The drug contains fifty to seventy three ingredients and was an example of practive of Polypharmacy.

DIOSCORIDES: He was a Greek army surgeon of Nero (54-68 A.D.). Due to his service opportunity of travelling many places. He studied many plants and became the originator of Materia Medica, which contained description of 600 plants and plant principles, of which 149 of these were already known to Hippocrates and not less than 90 are still used to-day.

ARETAEUS - Another follower of Hippocrates known as ARETAEUS, a talented physician who divides the diseases into (a) Acute diseases (b) Chronic diseases Acute diseases included. Pnuemonia, Pleurisy, Tetanus and Diphtheria, the chronic diseases included insanity, Paralysis and Phthisis. He was able to distinguish between the SPINAL and CEREBRAL PARALYSIS.

CELSUS— "DEMEDICINA"— An encyclopaedia of eight books written (A. D. 30) by a non medical man CELSUS. This book was printed in 1478, which seems to be FIRST MEDICAL BOOK PRINTED. This book mentioned four cardinal signs of inflammation of the medical students: CALOR, RUBOR, TUMOR, DOLOR: heat, redness, swelling, pain.

This book also gave description of diseases by anatomical divisions like—throat, throax, abdomen, feet. Hydrocephalus being the first and gout being the last. Volume—VII dealt extensively the surgical proceedures—methods of removal of arrow head, operations of Goitre, Hernia, lithotomy, couching for cataract and the most interesting Tonsillectomy by modern method of enaculeatia.

The period of Greek-Roman period of medicine reached its climax with the appearance of Galen.

GALEN (131-200 A.D.) was born at Pergamos in Asia Minor.

In practice, Galen followed the Hippocratic method accepting the doctrine of "HUMOURS", which regarded the body as composed of blood, phlegm, yellow bile and black bile; these nomenclatures were changed to sanguine, phlegmatic, melancholy and choleric after Galen in the mediaeval time.

He recognised the EXCITING and PREDISPOSING causes of diseases. He is said to be FIRST EXPERIMENTAL PHYSIOLOGIST. He recognised the value of Anatomy in the practice of medicine. All his knowledges were based on the dissection of apes and pigs, as dissection on human body was illegal. From the knowledge of dissected apes he was able to draw a certain amount of good description of Human skeleton and muscles and also the seven pairs of cranial nerves, the first pair OPTIC and the fifth the Facial. He distinguished between the SENSORY and MOTOR nerve and also the SYMPATHETIC nervous system.

He elaborated a system of pathology which combined the humoral ideas of Hippocrates with pythogorean theory of four elements and his own conception of a spirit or "PNEUMA" pertaining to all the parts.

Galen divided diseases into three classes:

(a) Those affecting similar parts or simple tissue (muscle, nerve),

(b) Organic (affecting compound tissue), (c) General or humoral i.e. dyscrasias organic diseases comprises malformations and abnormalities of size, position, and number of causes of diseases are: (a) Procatartic or exciting (b) Proegumenic or predisposing and synectic or coincident.

Symptoms follow the disease as shadow follows the substance.

He was a voluminous ancient writer and the greatest of the theorists and sytematists. He wrote 9 books on Anatomy, 17 on Physiology, 6 on Pathology, 16 essays on Pulse, 14 books on Megatechne or therapeutics (Ars, Magna)3 books on Temperament, 30 books on Pharmacy.

He also demonstrated that aphonia may be produced by the dissection of RECURRENT LARYNGEAL NERVE and also demonstrated the position of URETER. But he had certain misconception, specially the sources of blood and its circulation.

In the opinion of Galen the "VITAL PRINCIPLE" was the "PNEUMA" which entered the lung in the act of breathing and there mingled with blood. The blood was formed in the liver from the foodstuff of chyle, brought thence from the intestine by the portal vein. In the liver, the blood endowed with Natural spirit passed to the right ventricle, when it was distributed to nourish all the tissues and organs and also to the lungs in order that the impurities might be exhaled in the breath, part of the venous blood on reaching the heart, passed through minute and invisible pores in the interventricular septum and mingling with blood which arrived from the lungs by the arterial vein" (as he calls the pulmonary artery) became charged with a secored variety of Pheuma, the vital spirit.

Galen recognised that the arteries contained blood and not merely air, as had been belived before his days. He recognised that the heat that sets the blood in motion. But he had no idea that the blood circulated, he imagined that it ebbed and flowed in the vessels and his idea of a porous septum in the heart which was one of these fallacies which was blindly accepted and followed for centuries until the wrong ideas where detected.

Fortunately the Roman Emperor had high cultural values. They werew not utilising the terminology " public Hygiene" had nice system of water supply (100 gallons per head), sanitation, public bath etc.

After the fall of Greeks and Romans the ideas and practice of medicine were predominated by galilian thought and some persons or monks in the Arabian period were also followers of this principle.

Medicine in 15th and 16th century was the beginning of the renaissance period. The revolutionary ideas were though limited yet it was an attempt to escape from the tyranny and the then traditional limitations of churches and the dogmatic thought or influences of Roman's and Greece Medicine.

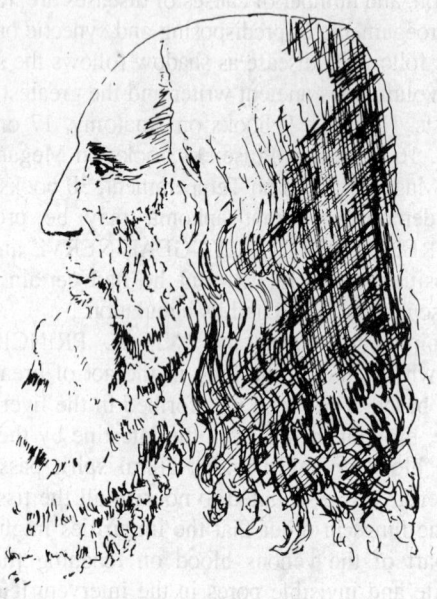

Fig. 6   LEONARDO DA VINCI (1452-1519)

LEONARDO DA VINCI (1452-1519): He was orginally a god–gifted artist. His appreciation of naturalism and deep in–sight made him to contribute remarkable drawings of human anatomical pictures.

He was first to demonstrate the ventricles of the brain by wax injection, and to depict correctly the foetus and its membrane within the uterus.

Originally he engaged to study the bones and muscles in relation to art and pursued his investigation to study the deeper parts of the body, visceres, brains, blood vessels and more specially the heart.

Remarkable were his studies of the bones, the skull, the spine, the Valves, muscles and vessels of the heart and also his discovery of the atrioventricular band in the right heart, his cross section of the brain and casts of its ventricles. Some of his notations about the origin and insetion of the museles were too minute.

ANDREAS VASALIUS—(1514-1564)

He belonged to a medical family. His father was a apothecary but

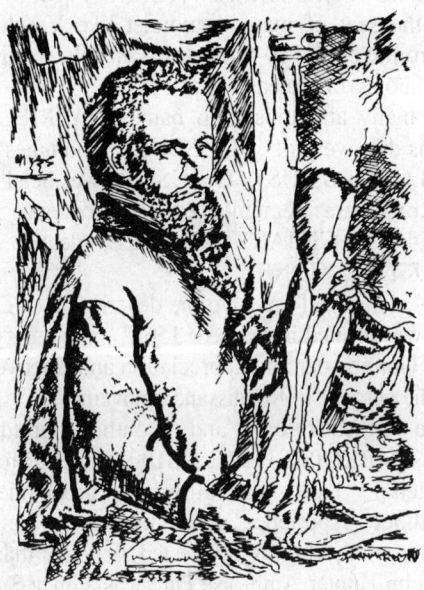

Fig. 7   ANDREAS VESALIUS (1514-1564)

his grandfather, great grandfather and great-great-grandfather were medical men of good outstanding. He secretly collected a skeleton of a criminal from a gallows from outside the city wall. It helped him in his studies. He was a professor of Surgery and Anatomy at PADUA in 1537.

Defying the Galen's authority, he published large plates of anatomical drawings known as "TABULA ANATOMICAE". The figures of the skeleton and the muscles were of great artistic value; many figures represented body in action. Vasalius corrected in showing that the lower jaw consisted of a single bone and the sternum was composed only three parts, not seven. He observed the valves of the vein and each artery supplying a viscus is accompained by a vein. In the first edition of his book he admitted the existence of minute "Pores" in the inter-venticular septum but in 1555 ultimately admitted that there were no pores and the blood cannot pass directly from one ventricle to the other, which in the later year hepled HARVEY to the discovery of circulation of blood. He also reflected certain lights in anthropology by observing that Germans are round headed and Belgians are long headed.

Vasalius was succeeded by REALDUS COLUMBUS (1510-1599) who succeeded in demonstrating PULMONARY CIRCULATION. It was published in his book DERE ANATOMICA in 1557.

Padua was the seat of many anatomist like Vaselius, Columbus, COITER of Groningen (1510-80) who was able to give a complete picture of the anatomy of the ear.

Among the many anatomist two names GABRIEL FALLOPIUS (1526-62) for his discovery of "AQUEDUCT" and tubes which bear his name, BARTOLOMEUS EUSTACHIUS who was head of the Dept. of anatomy at Rome are remembered for accurate illustration of THORACIC DUCT, CILIARY MUSCLE, details of FASCIAL MUSCLES, LARYNX, KIDNEY.

Tabulae of Vaselius did not give the description of EUSTACHIAN TUBES, which was printed in the year 1563.

Invention of Gunpowder and appreciation and discovery of practical anatomy drew the surgery in Renaissance movement.

In reality the surgical reforms and revolution started in Nineteenth century yet the AMBROISE PARE (1510-90) is still remembered for his surgical attempts and contribution. He proclaimed that "Mere knowledge without experience does not give the surgeon self confidence"—A remedy thoroughly tested is better than one recently invented. Like John Hunter Ambroise Pare was a great Surgeon.

His service to surgery did not merely concern gunshot wounds. He discussed in detail the treatment of fractures and dislocations. He suggested that syphilis was a course of Aneurysm and invented artery forceps and many other instruments.

As early as the Fourteenth century, the barber surgeons of England were organised in groups or GILDS. Every town of importance had its guild and it is estimated that there were about twenty or thirty such guilds. Very little was known about the details. From the Sixteenth century records were available. In this respect the name of THOMAS VICARY (1495-1561) is memorable for two reasons. He was the author and he was the first master of the united company of Barber's Surgeon and rapidly became the chief to the king Henry VIII. His book is titled as "A Treasure for Englishmen", containing the Anatomic of Man's body.

Among many others the following persons are still remembered.

(1) PIERRE FRANCO (1505-70)
    He was the first person to perform a suprapubic lithotomy. He wrote an article on HERNIA and described an operation on Strangulated Hernia. He had great success on operations on cataract.
(2) The name of two brothers FREE JACQUES and FRERE JEAN who practised surgery with greater success in lithotomy.

Glimpses of History of Medicine

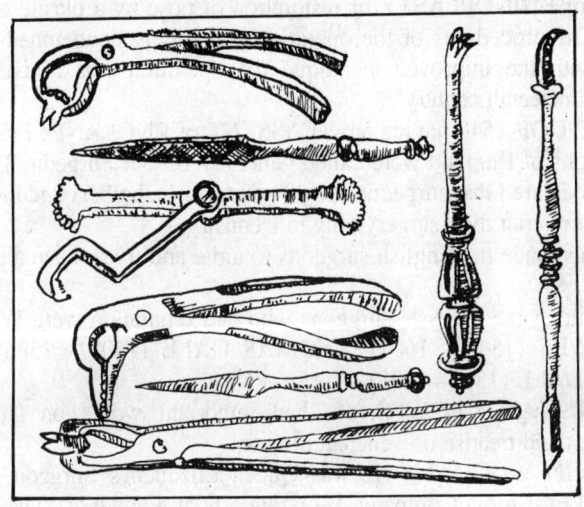

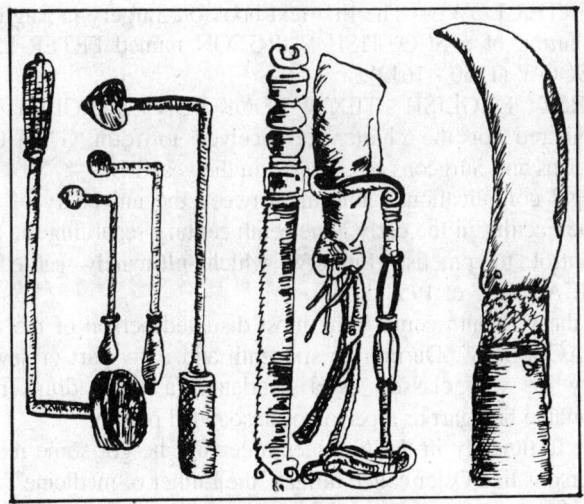

16TH CENTURY SURGERY.

Fig. 8   Dental Forceps to pull out teeth and file teeth.
Fig. 8.a   Amputation set and canters actual for extirpation.
          A Discourse of the whole art of chyrurgery by Peterzowe 4th. editon 1954.

(3) GASPARE TAGLIACOZZI: An Italian surgeon was remembered for RHINOPLASTY or restoration of nose by a plastic operation. The procedures of the operation was highly condemned later on; with the improved technique the operation was revived in the Nineteenth century.

ACT OF 1540 having Royal ASSENT of ENGLAND: Prior to this surgeons of England were called generally Barber Surgeon. The act of 1540 declared that surgeons should no longer be barbers and the barbers should restrict their surgery only to Dentistry.

This made the English surgeons to unite and try to have a corporate body.

Among the English Surgeons who had reputation were WILLIAM CLOWES (1540 - 1604); THOMAS GALE (1507 - 1586), JOHN WOODALL (1569 - 1643)

WILLIAM CLOWES: He had important works on Gun shoot wounds and treatise on venereal diseases.

JOHN WOODALI: He was Queen Elizabeth's Surgeon and also served East India Company. He wrote a book known as "The Pathway to the Surgeon's Chest", which gives details of the necessary instruments and equipments and how to use them.

PERTER LOWE—The first text book on Surgery in English was a contribution of a SCOTTISH SURGEON named PETER LOWE of GLASGOW (1550 - 1612).

FIRST ENGLISH TEXT BOOK ON SURGERY: He is remembered for the charter he received to form GACULTY OF Physicians and Surgeons of Glasgow in the year 1599.

Legal complications came up between the university of Glasgow and the Faculty in the early Nineteenth century regarding the authority to control to practise Surgery, which ultimately settled up by MEDICAL ACT of 1958.

In the sixteenth century the most disputed person of the time was "PARACELSUS". During the sixteenth and early part of seventeenth century he was classed as a charlatan, a mere drunken quack, disreputable braggart or a person of unsounded person.

But fortunately in the Nineteenth century he got some recognition and persons like Osler called him as "the Luther of medicine", Garrison called him "the most original thinker of the Sixteenth century.

The complexity of the theories of the Paracelsus was misunderstood or it was difficult to understand, made it so unpopular during his time.

PHILIPPUS AUREOLUS THEOPHRASTUS BOBBASTUS VON HOHNHEIM was known as PARACELSUS (1490-1541). He was born at Einsiedeln near Zurich. His father was a country doctor, latter a town

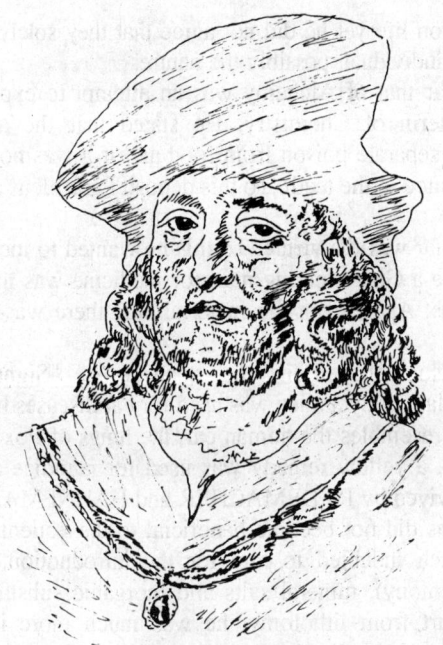

Fig. 9 Paracelsus (1493-1541).

physician. He married the matron of local pilgrim Hospital. In the early life he was attracted to mineralogy (lead mines) and in chemistry (Laboratory assistant). He travelled throughout Europe.

In 1526 he was appointed town physician at Basel and lecturer of medicine in the university. He was a voluminous writer but all his writings were published after his death. He himself predicted that his writings may be understasd twenty years after his death.

Paracelsus was a advocater of "Chemical view of life". In his principal work which he called as "PARAMIRUM", SULPHUR, MERCURY, SALT. Sulphur burns, mercury becomes smoke and salt becomes ash. Every action of the body depends on the proportions and actions of these principles. All diseases depend upon the result of maladjustment of the three.

Therefore there were THREE DISEASES and THREE REMEDIES.

In the present day it is a foolish talk but the good thing of the principal was that he tried to SIMPLIFY the PRESCRIPTION.

Another Paracelsus's teaching was that all medicines rest upon Four pillars or columns—Philosophy, astronomy, alchemy and virtue.

By philosophy he implied knowledge of natural phenomena; the astrology was not the astrology of the time. Though the stars have certain influence on life yet he did not agree that they solely controlled the destiny of an individual, possibly the nature.

The third pillar that of Alchemy was an attempt to explain health and disease in term of Chemistry. He stated that the aim of the alchemist was to separate poison from food and if it was not done, the poison was deposited in the teeth. To this deposit Paracelcus applied the name "Tartar".

The fourth pillar was the virtue. To this he wanted to mean that the physician must be a God—fearing man for medicine was more than a collection of facts. Apart from the material side there was a spiritual side.

Paracelsus also believed in the doctrine of "Signatures" or "Similars". The plant of cyclamen was used for ear diseases because the leaf of cyclamen resembles the human ear, the lungs of Fox were used for lung diseases, a yellow remedy was used for jaundice and so on. This view was revived by RADEMACHER and HAHNEMANN.

But those ideas did not become beneficial to the patients. Medical profession is much indebted to him for the introduction of certain metals (iron, antimony), mineral salts and inorganic substance in the therapeutics. Apart from lithotomy, he was much more inclined to nature's method of healing wounds with a Natural "balsam" manufactured by the body.

During this period JEROME CARDAN (1501-1576) was born in Milar though he had achieved much fame in medicine but his contribution in mathematics was much more. He wrote a book of algebra which is called "The book of great Art". It was said he discovered the rule of solving cubic equation. Though this was really discovered by a rival mathematician named TARTAGTA, it is still known as Cardan's rule. A book of very different nature was written by him on the significance of lines on the forehead An fantastic subjects of investigation Cardan's most popular work was DE SUBTILITATE 9(1551) a sort of household encyclopaedia, dealing all manner of subjects such as the marking of household linen, the raising of sunken slips, the identification of mushrooms, the origin of mountains, the twinkliing of stars, signalling by torches and the universal joint now known as the "Cardan shift".

A little book of precepts was written by him for the benefit of the children, known as "Praeceptorum Fillis liber" which contained sound advice like" Never associate with a stranger on a public road, "When you talk with a bad or dishonest man look at his hand not at his face", "Do not talk to other people of your self, your children, or your wife. He observed on things supernatural like dreams and omens.

SYPHILIS

Plagues and other epidemics had disastrous effects on mankind yet it acted as a stimulus to the medical profession to find out the causes and how to get rid of it. When in 1495 Charles VII of France conquered Naples, there broke-out a new and dreadful disease consisting of widespread skin eruption and ulceration with destruction of all the tissues causing many death and complication or other symptoms syndrome continued for long years to those who survived. The spanish occupants of Naples were infected by the sailors of Christopher columbus. They acquired the disease in the West Indies.

The French called it the "Naplian Disease" the Sapniarde called it the "French Disease". While FRACASTORIUS was the first person to call it "SYPHILIS" which still remains to-day.

Whether the disease was known before or not, it is not known to any body but some of the ancient mythological writings had given a picture, which is similar to syphilis. But the epidemic form which broke out in Naples was unparallel in the history.

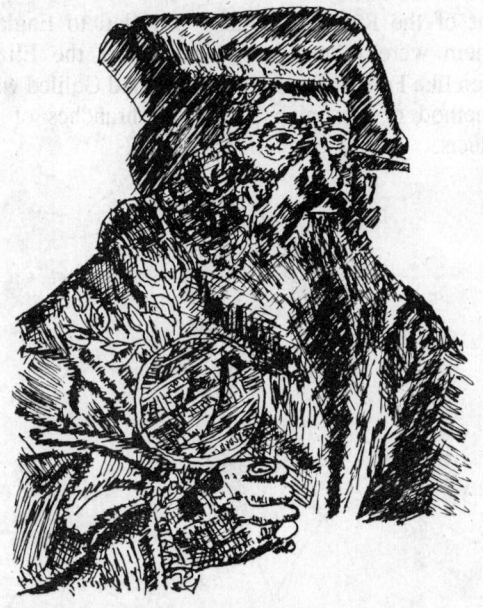

Fig. 10 GIROLAMO FRACASTORO (1484-1553).

HIERONYMUS FRACASTORIUS GIROLAMO (1484-1553) was born at Yerona. He wrote a poem in 1521 called "that Divine poem". It was entitled "SYPHILIS, SIVE MORBUS GALLICUS published in

1530.

The poem also indicated Mercury and Guacum or Holy Wood a remedy of American origin.

Though Bacteria was not known during Fracastorius time, yet his observation had made us to call him as "FOUNDER OF MODERN EPIDEMIOLOGY".

TYPHUS

He was among the first to recognise TYPHUS FEVER. In 1546, he published the great work, DE CONTAGIONE in which he described the three methods of infection:

(a) Infection by direct contact.

(b) Infection by "Fomites" a word which he was the first to apply to infected clothing, utensils etc. and infection at a distance, as in small pox or plague.

(c) He presumed the existence of imperceptibly particles or "Seminaria", the Seeds of Diseases which multiply rapidly and propagate similar to each other.

The light of the Renaissance also travelled to England. Though many of them were followers of Galen. Yet the Elizabethan era produced men like Francis Bacon, Descartes and Galiled who with their inductive method of reasoning guided all branches of science into fruitful products.

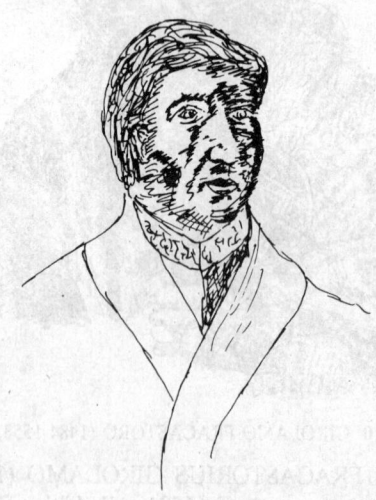

Fig. 11 THOMAS LINACRE M.D. (1460-1524)

English physicians headed by THOMAS LINACRE (1460-1524) obtained from the king Henry VIII letters of permission to form a corporated body of Physicians in the year 1518, which became the ROYAL COLLEGE OF PHYSICIAN. This body was empowered to decide who should practice within the city or within a radius of seven miles around it and also to examine and to issue licence to practise throughout the kingdom except those medical graduates of Oxford and Cambridge. The college was given the authority to examine the prescription and medical drugs shops (apothecaries); and to impose fine for any default and if necessary imprisonment.

The first president of the Royal College of Physician was Dr. THOMAS LINACRE.

A sister university of Cambridge was also formed and claimed distinguised physicians like:

Dr. JOHN CAIUS who succeeded Dr. Lincre in the presidentship.

Dr. Caius contributed a detail account of an epidemic disease.

Known as "SWEAT SICKNESS".

This epidemic of "Sweat Sickness" was very devastating and was mostly among the soldiers of Henry VIII Earl of Richmond.

Henry VIII had a great victory in the battle of Bosworth and planning a coronation but the devastation of Sweat Sickness was so great that he had to postpone the ceremony. This reappeared again in 1508, 1517, 1551. This type of epidemic also occurred in France 1718.

The disease began very suddenly with shivering and violent fever, headache, lethargy, abdominal pain and profuse perspiration. It lasted only for twenty four hours, but many died within the day and some within the first hours of attack. There was a characteristic stains and vesicular rash. In "History of Eidemics in Britain" quotes a contemporary description of the symptoms as" a grete sweating and shynking with redness of the face and body and a contiunued thirst with a great heat and headeche because of the fumes and venoms.

During this period English medical books were printed on which a book known as "THE BOOK OF CHILDREN" on Pediatric was printed by THOMAS PHAYRE and an English translation on midwifery.

But in reality the renaissance to Britain was brought by WILLIAM HARVEY who not only solved the problem of Blood circulation and original contribution to British midwifery.

The Seventeenth century was a period of great intellectual activity and in the field of medicine it was a golden age.

The name of FRANCIS BACON, Lord Verulam (1561-1626) and DESCARTES, greatests philosopher of 17th century made much contribution in the field of philosophy.

The uprise of the Philosophical thoughts went side by side with medicine. Medical professional people got attracted with the thoughts of reasoning in their deductions. Francis Bacon has often been compared with Roger Bacon (1214-1294).

Both of them favoured experiment as opposed to argument. They inspired men to think for themselves and to make experiments and to hold past to facts. To them truth was derived from experience, he (Francis Bacon) lead no new school of Philosophy. He simply revived the Platonic method of reasoning in his book "NOVUM ORGANUM" (1620) he asked men to leave and not to worship the then four popular thoughts (accepted authority, popular opinion, legal bias, personal prejudice and to replace them by the "inductive" method of reasoning based upon experience. Bacon was the father of objective and realistic tradition in modern philosophy while Descartes was the father of the subjective and idealistic tradition in modern philosophy.

Though he had not made much reference of Roger Bacon, yet men of Science and Scientific reasonings had recognised Roger Bacon long after his death.

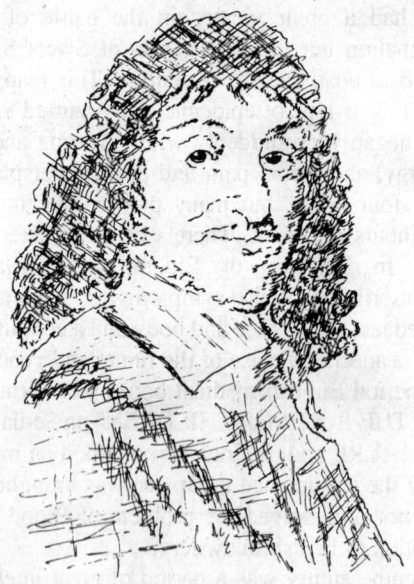

Fig. 12 RENE DESCARTES (1596-1650).

RENE DESCARTES (1596-1650) was a French philosopher. He wrote the first book of physiology. He spent much part of his life in

Holland. The effect of "CARTESIAN" philosophy was considerable on medical science. The central idea in his philosophy was that mind and matter constitued the universe, but that there was no connection between them. He conveived "SOUL" was lying in the pineal body.

Man was nothing but a machine made by God. Animal did not possess mind and soul. Man although a machine possessed mind which acted upon the body. The proof of existence of mind was conscious thought. He wrote that except of our own thoughts there was nothing in our power. His conception made great influence on medical progress. His conception attracted to the school of "IATRO-PHYSICISTS" who regarded human body as a mechanical contrivance.

During this period there appeared a versatile Italian, named as GALILEO GALILEI (1564-1642).

He studied medicine also. In the church he watched the movement of a swinging lamp and compared it with the beat of his own pulse, which inspired him to use it for recording time. He invented the pendulum and telescope. The relation between mechanics and measurement, stressed by Galileo, had accelerated to many diagnosis in medicine.

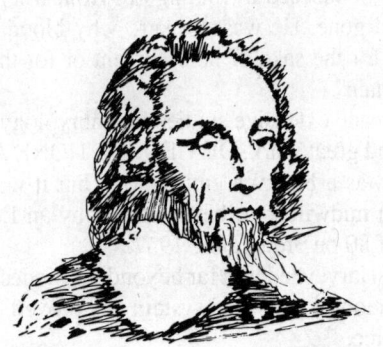

Fig. 13 WILLIAM HARVEY (1578-1657).

THERE came in the scene a person known as WILLIAM HARVEY (1578-1657) who revolutionized the medical science, and changed the entire out-look and laid the foundation of the modern medical practice. He was born at Folkestone. After getting his primary education at Canterbery and Caius College Cambridge he got his M.D. in 1602 at

PADUA. After finishing his medical career in Padua he started practice in England and became the fellow of the Royal College of Physician. He said that "The movement of the blood is constantly in a circle and is brought about by the beat of the heart".

After twelve years of his discovery he published in 1628 a book known as "Exercitatio Anatomica De Motu cordis et Sanguinis in Animalibus".

He had keen interest in comparative anatomy. He observed that the movement of heart could be observed more readily in cold-blooded animals like frogs and fishes. Fortunately he was permitted to conduct post-mortem examination. A person named as Thomas Parr died at the alleged age of 153 years. King Charles ordered to find out the cause of his death: Harvey conducted a post-mortem and found that the death was due to pleuro-pneumonia. He also studied embryology which led him to publish his second work "DE GENERATIONE ANIMALIUM". He advanced the view that foetus assisted it s own delivery by active movement. The anatomical treatise on the movement of Heart and Blood in animal (DE MOTU CORDIS ET SANGUINIS) is probably the greatest book in medical literature. He showed that the Heart was a hollow muscular organ and the blood impelled into the arteries gave rise to pulse".

He made various experiments by ligaturing the various arteries and viens but could not succeed in finding out from where the blood came and where it had gone. He was not sure why blood circulates and he wrote "Whether for the sake of nourishment or for the communication of heat is not certain".

Hervey also made extensive studies in embryology which led him to publish his second great work, DE GENERATIONE ANIMALIUM" in 1651, though it was a book on embryology but it may be regarded as the first book on midwifery to be published by an English author. He died at the age of 80 on 3rd of June 1957.

The genius of Harvey led him far beyond his predecessors. He altered the entire conception of the blood system and proved the heart to be the central motive force.

He showed that the heart was a hollow muscle and that the blood impelled.

GASPARE ASELLI OF CREMONA (1581-1625)

He discovered the LACTEAL VESSELS and published a book on the subject "DE LACTEIS VEINS", a student of the Gaspare traced the entire course of the lacteals and a another student of Padua discovered the lymph vessels and the distinction between the lacteals and lymph.

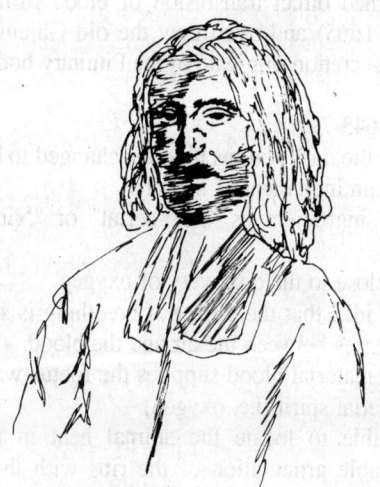

Fig. 14 MARCELLO MALPIGHI (1628-94).

Apparently Harvey did not accept the discovery. He only conceived some sort of channel between the smallest arteries and vein; with the introduction of Microscope MARCELLO MALPIGHI demonstrated a fine network of connecting vessels of the arteries and veins in the lung of a frog. Malpighi was also first to describe the layers of skin, lymph nodes of the spleen and the glomeruli of the kidney. A student of Malpighi ANTONIO VALSALV contributed much in the Anatomy and physiology of the ear.

A new epoch was ushered in another field of human knowledge in the chemistry by HON ROBERT BOYLE (1627-91). The potentiality of air was recognised by Boyle.

But the interaction of air and blood was not yet understood and the problem of respiration was solved by LOWER and MAYOW. Lower was able to denounce the misconception that the nasal mucous which accompanied a cold arises from the nasal membrane was from brain.

MAYOW was a lawyer and later on turned into medicine. His description of the mechanism the inspiratory movement accompanied by the diaphragm and intercostal muscles and the expiratory was only a movement holds good to-day.

RICHARD LOWER of Cornwall (1631-91) was an able physiologist and also a successful practitioner. He injected dark venous blood into the insufflated lungs and conducded that its consequent bright colour was due to the fact that it had obserbed some of the air passing through the lung.

He first performed direct transfusion of blood from are animal to another (February 1665) and overthrew the old Galenic and vesalices idea that the nasal secretion originate in the Pituitary body.

JOHNMAYOW (1643-79)

He showed that the dark venous blood is changed to bright red blood by taking up a certain ingredient of the air.

He termed the ingredient as "Neo-aerial" or "Nitro-aerial spirit" particles.

This was very close to the discovery of oxygen.

He grapsed the idea that the object of breathing is simply to course an interchange of gases between the air and the blood.

He son that the material blood supplies the foetus was not only food but also the nitro-aerial spirit (i.e. oxygen)

He was also able to locate the animal heat in the mascle. He discovered the double articulation of the ribs with the spine and the function of intercostal museler.

ZACHARIAS JANSEN MICROSCOPE

The microscope which enabled Malpighi to complete the work of Harvery was probably the ancients. Roger Bacon first suggested the use of lenses spectacles.

He also held the opinion that there must be some constitutent in the

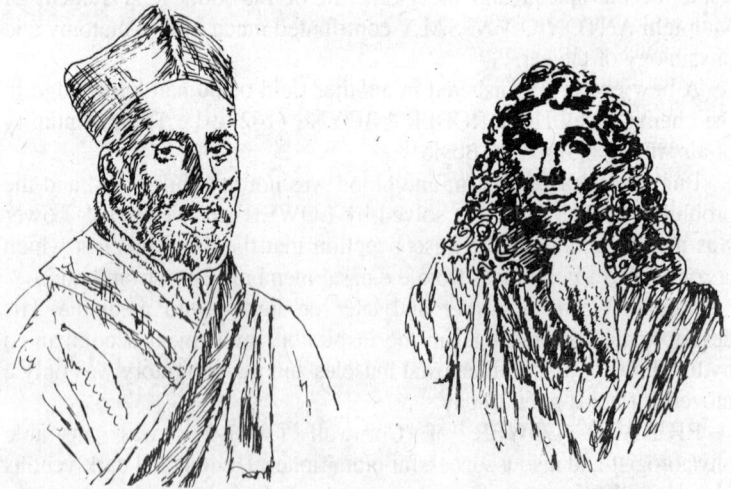

Fig. 15 ATHANASIUS KIRCHER (1602-80)

Fig. 16 Antonj van Leeuwenhoek (1632-1723)

air which was necessary for the stool.

It was ZACHARIAS JANSEN a spectacle maker of Middelburg in Holland who in the year 1609 accidently discovered the principle of the telescope and microscope by placing two lens together in a tube.

ANTONJ VAN LEEUWENHOEK (1632-1723)

A merchant of Delft, was early inventor of microscope. He with his own prepared lens was able to have a magnification of 160 times.

ANTHANASIUS KIRCHER (1602-80)— A professor of physiology at Wurzburg was possibly the first person to apply microscope to the study of disease. He saw countless small worms in the blood of plague stricken patients. They were really not the plague bacilli but masses of red blood cells, but he was confident that contagious diseases were conveyed by minute living organism.

In the field of biology the earliest and most briliant worker was ROBERT HOOKE (1635-1703). Many of his biological drawings of insects and plants have been reproduced as standard illustration.

Another pioneer in the field of microscope was also a DUTCHMAN (JAN SWAMMERDAM-1637-80)

He made wonderful drawings on insect and dragonflies.

Swammerdan's best work was "ALIIS INSERVIENDO CONSUMOR" or History of insects (1669).

He gave accurate like histories with finner anatomy of the bees, the magtlies, the snarl, the clam, the sqid, the frog. He was the first to discern and discrible the red blood corpuscles (1658), discovers the values of the lymphaties (1664) and discovered the medico legal fact that the foetal lungs will float after respiration has taken place (1667).

LEYDEN was a another centre of learning in the 16th century. Among the many learned person who had the training from there FRANCIS DE LA BOE or SYLVIUS (1614-72) was one of them, who discovered FISSURE OF SYLVIUS in the brain; another GOVERT BIDLOO (1649-1713), who dissected sixty dead bodies and was poineer in Anthropology; described in his treatise on obsteology the difference in the cranium of the different races of mankind.

Anatomy flourished exceedingly in many other countries during this century. The names of BARTHOLIN, STENSEN, WIRSUNG, BRUNNER, PACCHIONI, PEYER, VIEUWSSENS, WARTON, MEIBOM, SCHNEIDER, are remembered by the reader Anatomy, Certain duct a gland, or some other structure are named from the discoverer.

REGNIER DE GRAAF a Dutch physiologist discovered the "Graafian Follices": or the ovary made important observations on saliva

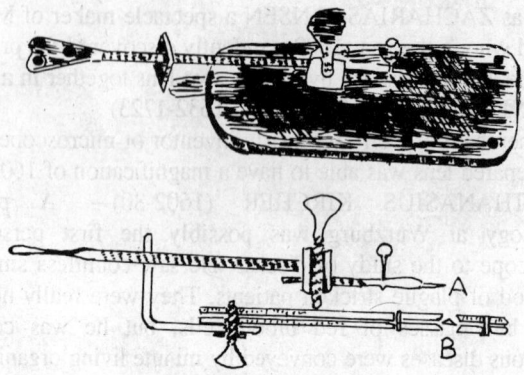

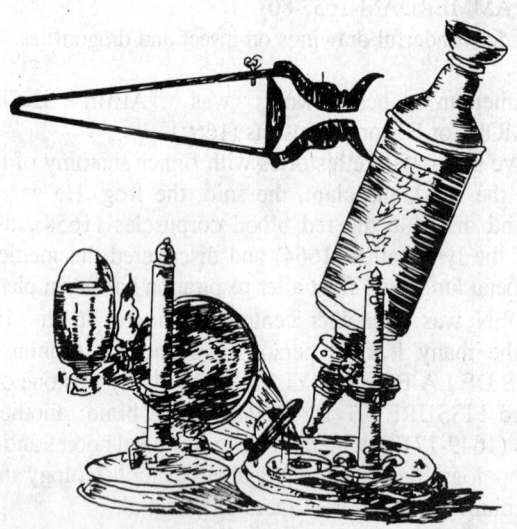

Fig. 17   Leeuwenhoek's microscope. The object to the examined, mounted on holder A, may be moved in two directions by screw adjustments so as to bring it within focus of the small lens B, which is firmly fixed between two perforated brass plates.

Fig.17.a   Robert Hooke's microscope, from his Micrographia, 1665. The objective is a tiny double convex lens of short focus, mounted in a cell close to a pin-hole diaphragm. A wider field might be secured by a plano-convex lens within the tube at fixed distance from the eye. Hooke often dispensed with this.

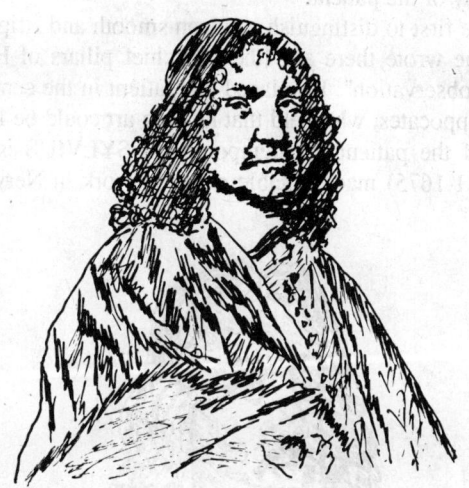

Fig. 18 FRANCISCUS SYLVIUS (1614-72)

and bile, whereas HENDRIK VAN DEVENTER studied the variation on female pelvis and their effects on labour.

TREND in medicine:

In the beginning of the 17th century two curious trends in medicine came up one School regarded the body as a machine and tried to explain that all the working of the body whether in health or disease as a Physical or mechanical in nature. This was the "IATRO-PHYSICAL or IATRO-MECHANICAL" theory.

Another explained life as a chemical process and all its working are action or the reaction of some chemical components.

This was known as "IATRO-CHEMICAL".

Descartes upheld the Iatro-physical theory, but primarily he was a Philosopher of deductive method of reasoning and incidentally a Physiologist.

In this period there were certain people who highly advocated the "Itro-physical" theory yet they contributed their best in certain field of medicines.

SANCTORIUS (1561-1636) was among them. He first invented the clinical thermometer, trocar and cannula, and Pulse clock. Similarly GIOVANI ALPHONSO BORELLI, an Italian, was a staunch follower of the Itro-physical thoughts; GIORGIO BAGLIVI, a physicist, a brilliant clinician found that every thing could not be explained in the term of Physics as such he said that the healing art could be learned only by a study of the patient.

He was the first to distinguish between smooth and striped muscles. In his book he wrote there are "the two chief pillars of Physick" are "Reason and observation". He placed the patient in the centre as a true disciple of Hippocates, who held that healing art could be learned only by a study of the patient. Contemporary to SYLVIUS is THOMAS WILLIS (1621-1675) made notable research work in Nervous system

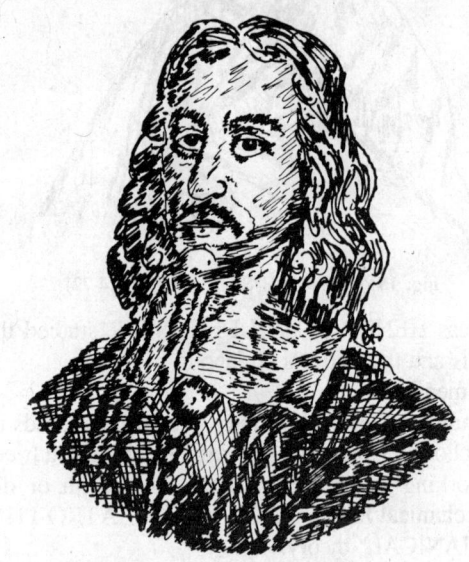

Fig. 19 THOMAS WILLIS (1621-75)

and gave a fine description of Brain. His name is still remembered today when one thinks "CHRLE OF WILLIS" and "PARACUSIS OF WILLIS". He is also credited with the discovery of the presence of Sugar Diabeticusine.

A distinguished contemporary of Wills was FRANCIS GLISSON. In his book "ANATOMIA HEPATIS" he gave the accurate description of the capsule of the liver and his article DE RACHITIDE (1650) was a classical account of infantile rickets.

There were three great clinical physicians in the 17th century. They were "GLISSON", "MAYERNE", "SYDENHAM", MAYERNE, SIR THEODORE TURQUET of MAYERNE (1473-1655) was a careful observer and an eminent physician. He introduced calomel and of Mercurial lotion known as "black wash".

The latter half of the 17th century marked the advent of THOMAS SYDENHAM (1624-89) in the field of medicine who was rightly styled as English Hippocrates.

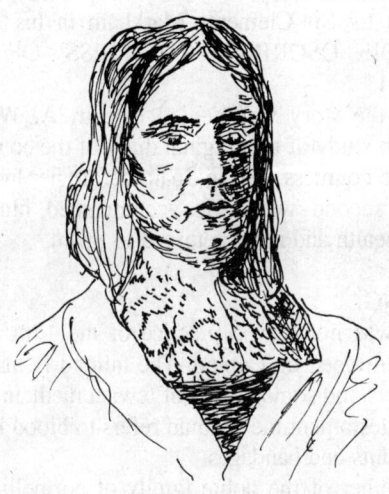

Fig. 20 THOMAS SYDENHAM (1624-89)

He was born at Wynoford Engle in Dorset, graduating at Oxford; Sydenham continued his medical studies at Montpellier.

Sydenham was essentially a clinician, he rejected entirely the Iatrophysics or Iatro-chemistry theories. His method consisted in the careful observation and recording the phenomena of disease. He had the greatest regard with respect to the Hippocratic outlook. In therapeutics he preferred simple remedies.

He treated fever by cooling method, phthisis by open air exercise, anaemia with iron, syphilis with mercurial preparation until free salivation occured. He popularised the use of quinine yielding cinchona bark lately introduced from Peru in the treatment of Malaria. He tried to impress upon the medical profession the necessity of discovering specifics for disease condition. He belonged to that group who wanted to follow Hippocrates, to observe and follow nature either assisting the nature to open the pathway or to attack the malady directly with specific than the other group who disbelieved the existence and efficacy of specific which could not be explained by the laws.

The romantic tale of the discovery of Cinchona is very familiar to every student of medicine. Early in the 17th century, the countess of Cinchon, wife of the viceroy of Peru was cured of a fever by the use of a remedy suggested by a local governor, a powder prepared from the bark of a tree which came to be known as countess's powder. She distributed a large quantities of the bark to the citizens of Lima, later introduced in Spain. This story was recorded by sebastian Bado in 1663 and was repeated by Sir Clements Markham in his "MEMOIR OF LADY ANA DE OSORINO, COUNTESS OF CHINCHON, LONDON, in 1874."

Unfortunately the story was denied by Mr. A. W. Haggis, who during the research study of the original diary of the count of Chinchon has proved that the countess died in Spain before her husband was sent to Peru and his second wife who accompanied him in Peru, led remarkably good health and never returned to Spain.

BLOOD-LETTING

Blood letting was not only a practice of the 17th country of this procedure was mentioned in Talmud. The talmud is mainly a book of regulations and laws and some details of fewish medicine which are not to be found in old testament the Talmud refers to blood letting, cupping and the case of splints and bandages.

CELUS, a member of the noble family of cormelli, wrote a book known as "DE MEDICINA". It was an every clopaedia written in 30 A.D. Blood letting as a means of therapeuties aid was also mentioned venesection also mentioned in the gnueo-Roman period. The followers of school of salerno advocated the method, referance of which are found in the book named "Passionarius" written by "GARIOPONTUS (d-1050).

The followers of the school of salerna had high superstition of venesection. The technique of venesection was fully described in the "Regimen". One of which was said in a poem.

"Three special months September, April, May; There are in which 'tis good to ope a vein; In there three months the moon bears greatest sway".

The mediaeval period of medicine is regarded as an age of decadence and of stagnation the very name "mediaeval" implies the negation of progress and suggests backwardness, superstition and sloth conception of disease war archaie, diagnosis and progresis were based mainly an stars and on the inspection of wine of some herbs which nature were illunderstood.

At the same it was also deplored by certain section of the people like Guido han pranchs (1115) of Paris.

During the black-death epidemic (plegue) of 1348 the seashore of North Sea, Mediterranean, Central Asia, Italy, France, England and Russia patients were advised blood lettings and drinking vinigar.

In the 15th century familiar illustration of 28 veins were shown from where the matria Pcecans (ie noxious object is moving).

It was PIERE BRISTON (1478-1522) of Paris who painted act that the contrary method of "derivation" used by Hippocrates consisting in blood-letting near the lesion and on the same side, was to be preferred. But gradually when in the 19th century and the later part of the 18th century of disease changed. Blood letting was denamed.

18th CENTURY MEDICINE

After Sydenham the master clinician there emerge innumerable theorists and speculators in the field of medicine. Practically the whole of 18th century in Europe was marked by plethora of theories and hypotheses concerning the cause of diseases and consequently the methods of therapeutics and practice were numerous and diverse.

This was the condition of affiars at about the beginning of the century when two great scientists supplied the need of the age. To the the apparent choas NEWTON applied law and LINNAEUS brought order. In the medicine the outstanding figure was Neuton's Principia was published in 1687. BOERHAAVE, one of the most eminent physician of all times.

SIR ISAAC NEWTON (1642-1727): Everyhody knows about him.

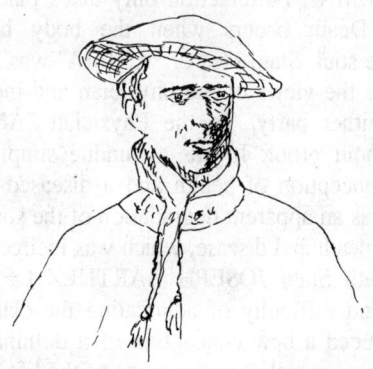

Fig. 21 CARL VON LINNE (1707-78)

Though he was not concerned directly with medicine, yet it was bound to exercise a profound effect upon all science.

At a slightly later date carl von Linne known as LINNAEUS (1707-78) a successful physician as well as one of the greatest botanist of all times introduced the binomial method of classifying plants, having its genus and species. It gave science a means of classification and to bring order and uniformity in place of confusion and diversity. The SYSTEMA NATURAE was published in 1773 and ultimately the method of classification extended to animals (Homo Sapiens).

Many other theories and speculations extended at about this time, but they all became obsolete, but as they played some part in the path of evolution, some reference of the sponsorers and their theories must be made.

GEORG ERNST STAHL (1660-1734)

The conflict and compromise between medicine and religion is seen throughout this age and is the most interesting part in the history of medicine. Medical professional people were occasionally the victim of the religious superstition in the 18th century unknowingly.

Medicine became so materialistic that the function of human body in health and disease were considered either a normality of Physics and chemistry or not; reaffirming the existence and importance of "SOUL" responsible for health and disease. Stahl was one of them who had firm conviction on "SOUL".

Stahl discarded Chemistry or Physics and he did not give much stress in Anatomy. He did not admit like Descartes that soul and body each went their separate way. In the opinion of Stahl soul and body were closely blended and the source of all vital movement was the "SOUL" or "ANIMA". Putrefaction only takes place after death in a soulless body. Death occurs when the body became unsuitable habitation for the soul. Stahl idea of "ANIMA" was not a new one. He tried to reconcile the views of the physician and theologicians but he could satisfy neither party. To the Physician "ANIMISM" was an idiotic idea without proof. It was an undue simplicity in matter of treatment and conception of health and a diseased condition. To the theologician it was an apparent degradation of the soul as a defender of the body against death and disease, which was ineffective.

After the death Stahl JOSEPH BARTHEZ OF MONTPELLIER (1734-1806) found difficulty of advocating the claim of "SOUL" or "BODY", introduced a new conception of a dominant force "VITAL PRINCIPLE". It was merely another name of the life–principle.

Associated with the name of Stahl is FRIEDRICH HOFFMAN

(1660-1742). Though he was born during Stahl's time, they had no common similarity. His system of medicine was based upon the belief that the universe was pervaded by a vital substance which is finer than all other matter but not exactly spirit, soul or mind and this fine delicate something maintained the body in a state of "TONIC" equilibrium. In Hoffman's view, disease resulted from excess or deficiency of tonus.

At the end of Hoffman's era JOHN BROWN, was born in Scotland (1735-88). He was a follower of Hoffman.

He was twice President of the Royal Medical Society; "BRUNONIAN system" of thought of the life was a controversial debates in the Royal Society between the students of Brown and Cullen.

The Brunonian system was very simple, life according to Brown depended upon continuous stimulation. The stimulants were warmth, food, muscular movement, intellectual energy, emotion etc. Disease was the result of excess or defect in the stimulation. Acting upon this assumption, Brown classified diseases into "ASTHENIC" and "STHENIC". The treatments were aimed to apply LARGE and HEROIC doses of medicine, specially stimulating drugs; the result was very adverse and death rolls were more than cure.

Violent controversy and criticism went very high up regarding the "LARGE and HEROIC" doses. God helped humanity from the horror of the use of large doses.

At the opposite a person known as "SAMUEL HAHNEMANN" (1755-1843) was born. In course of time he became renowned person and a Saviour of the ailing humanity by offering a new and an alternative method of treatment. Though people initially denied much of his theories but with the events of time and progress they gradually accepted. The world has accepted him and his methods.

Dr. F.C.S. Hahnemann was born on 10th April 1755 in the Electorate of Saxon in Germany. His father Christian Gottfried Hahnemann was a porelain painter. He spent several years in the public school of Meissen and ultimately in the university of Leipzig. After two years of study in the university, he left for Vienna, to have a wide experience under Quarin, to whom he was indebted much. On August 1779 he was awarded a degree of medicine at the university of Erlangen.

His thesis was "A summary of the condition of cramp according to cause and cure". Being a reputed translator and chemist in 1790 he was busy in translating a treatise on Materia Medica by Dr. William Cullen of Edinberg, a famous consultant and an authority of Materia Medica of the 18th century. Inquisitive mind of Hahnemann wanted to prove the truth in the Materia Medica of Cullen. He made trial of Cinchona bark

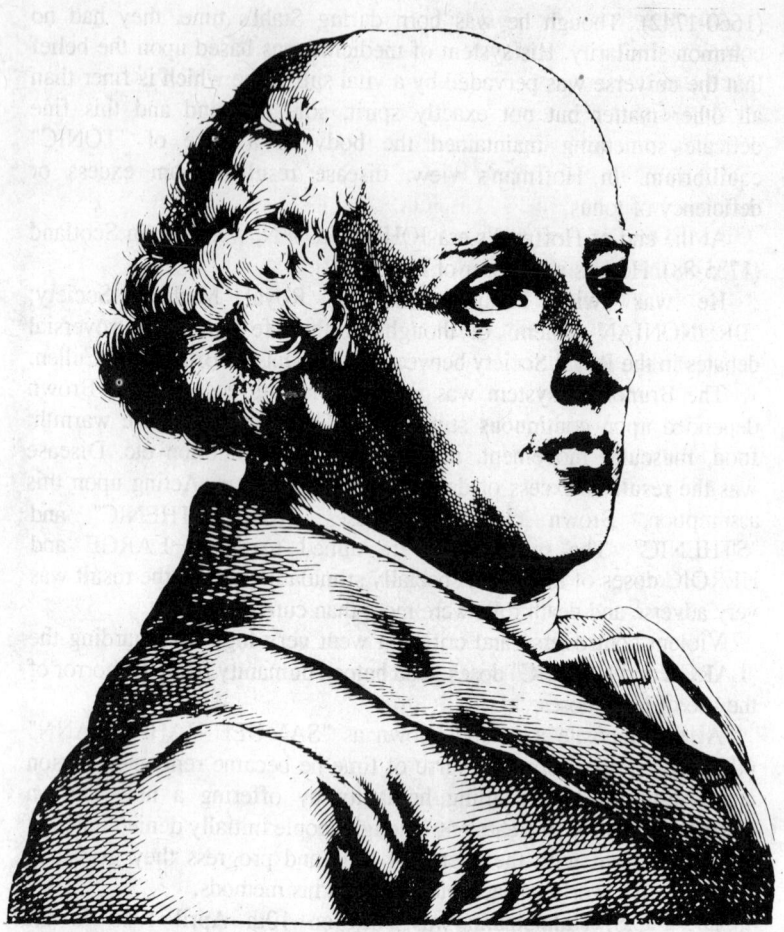

Samuel Christian Friedrich Hahnemann

on his own body in large doses, in consistence with the system of practice. The symptomatology of ague appeared in strong paroxysm. It inspired him to have experiment on his own body with other active substance. The result as expected was the same in each case with slight variation according to thier inherent reactive capacity. This made him to establish "HOMOEOPATHY". The chief principle of Homoeopathy lies in the infinitesimal dose, but in the selection of drugs according to the principle of "SIMILIA SIMILIBUS CURENTUR" "Let likes be treated by likes".

In other words durgs which, when administered to healthy persons cause certain symptoms are to be given in a diseased condition when such similar symptoms are present.

In the year 1796 in his essay on "new principles for ascertaining the curative of drugs" he put shape to his new method of curing the sick. In 1805 he published a book known as "Medicine of experience" which ultimately become in 1810 as "ORGANON OF RATIONAL SYSTEM OF MEDICINE," which was ultimately changed as "ORGANON OF MEDICINE". It has six editions. The remarkable contribution in the field of medicine is his theory of Chronic Diseases put in a treatise known "CHRONIC DISEASE" (1810).

The fundamentals of his new therapeutics are:
(1) Drug proving on healthy human being.
(2) The selection and administration of so proved medicines according to law of similars.
(3) Single remedy.
(4) Minimum dose.
(5) Theory of vital force.
(6) Theory of drug dynamisation to bring out the latent curative power of the drug.
(7) New conception of health, disease and cure.

There can be no doubt that, Hahnemann had added greatly to our knowledge of the action of drug.

The new idea was strenuously opposed by apothecaries, who were likely deprived of their profits and also by the dogmatist. The Empirics and methodists who were active in the 18th century revolted against Hahnemann, yet Homoeopathy gained popularity throughout the world for its efficacy and practised by many followers.

Before Hahnemann there was a famous clinical teacher of the century at LEYDEN, he was "HERMANN BOERHAAVE" (1668-1738). Prior to coming in medicine, he was put to theology. For twenty years he was the central figure of European medicine. Like Hippocrates he placed the patient in the centre of the picture and favoured more observation rather than argument.

His chief works are the "INSTITUTIONES MEDICAE" (1708) and "APHORISMI" (1709) both of which had many editions. The "INDEX PLANATRUM", 1710 is a catalouge of the Botanical Gardens of Leyden, which he betterly classified and enlarged: Not content with the reputation as a leading physician and botanist, he accepted the chair of Chemistry in 1718 and 1731.

During this contemporary period of Boerhaave there was another famous teacher known as "WILLIAM CULLEN" (1712-90). He was

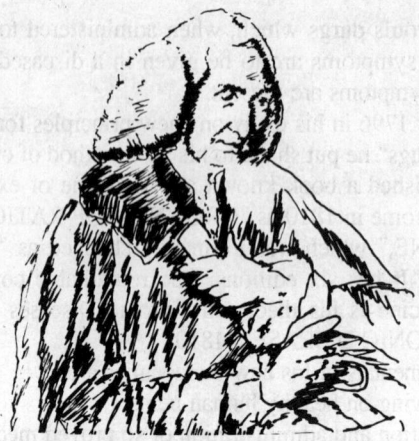

Fig. 22 WILLIAM CULLEN (1712-90)

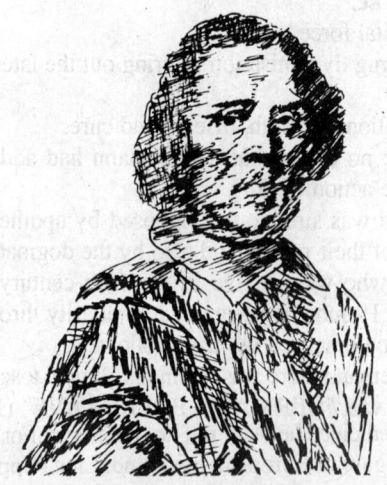

Fig. 23 HERMANN BOERHAAVE (1668-1738)

born at Hamilton in Lankashire. From the Grammar School of Hamilton Young Cullen proceeded to Glasgow University but as there was not yet any Medical faculty, he became an apprentice to a Surgeon and later to an apothecary in London. He had a good friendship with WILLIAM HUNTER. During his practice time, he was keen in lecturing not only in Chemistry, but also in Botany, Materia Medica and Physics. He is regarded as founder of Glasgow School of Medicine. At different time he had the privilege of occupying the highest chair of the Institution of Theory of Medicine and Professor of Medicine. He was the author of a textbook known as "FIRST LINES OF THE PRACTICE OF PHYSIC" and also of a treatise on Materia Medica.

Boerhaave and Cullen were two great teachers of 18th century, the former at the beginning and later toward the end.

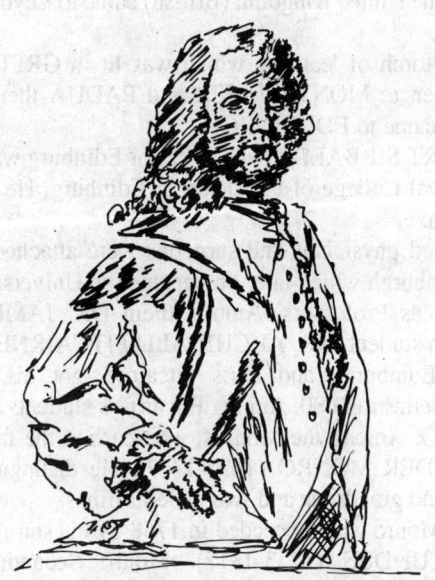

Fig. 24 ALBRECHT VON HALLER (1708-77)

Boerhaave had attracted many students to Leyden the then one of the best centre of learning, one of the most eminent was ALBRECHT VON HALLER (1708-77) of Berne. He is remembered as a poet, botanist and as a pioneer physiologist. One of his poetry "DIE ALPEN" was of high standard, a description of Swiss mountain; in the field of botany his work was on the FLORA OF SWITZERLAND. In the field of physiology his greatest achievement was his demonstration of the irritability of muscles and of the sensibility of nerve. He proved that irritability was an attribute of the muscle tissue, inherent in the muscle itself and not dependent upon the nerve supplying the nerve. GLISSION suggested the hypothesis but HALLER proved it by series of experiment upon excised muscle tissue.

His ELEMENTA PHYSIOLOGIAE in eight volumes (1759-66) was an immense work.

Another student of Boerhaave was GERHARD VAN SWIETEN

(1700-42) a roman catholic who was also a student of Leyden.

Being requested by the Empress Maria Theresa, he came to Vienna and reconstructed the Medical School of Vienna, which was later on taken by ANTON DE HAEN (1704-76)

Haen was the author of treatise on therapeutics in which he highly condemned the excess drugging which was prevalent at that time many students from the United Kingdom (British) came to Leyden for study of medicine.

In fact the torch of learning which was lit in GREECE passed to SALERNO, then to MONTPELLIER and PADUA then to LEYDEN and ultimately came to EDINBURGH.

SIR ROBERT SIBBALD (1641-1722) of Edinburg was famous as a founder of Royal College of Physician of Edinburg. He also spent ten years at Leyden.

Many reputed physicians and surgeons were attached to the Town College of Edinburgh which later on became the University. They were also appointed as Professors. Among them DR. JAMES HALKET, another Leyden student, DR. ARCHIBALD PITCAIRNE (1652-1713). a student of Edinburgh and Paris pitcairne. got his Doctorate of Medicine at Rheims in 1680. Among Pitcairne's students at Leyden was JOHN MONRO. Among the Monros, who carried the family tradition was ALEXANDER MONRO (1697-1767). He distinguished himself from his sons and grandsons and was called Primus.

Alexander Monro was succeeded in 1758 by his son ALEXANDER MONRO SECUNDUS (1733-1817). Monro Secundus was more brilliant than his father. It is said that during fifty years tenure in the chair about 40,000 students attended his classes.

He discovered the "FORAMEN OF MONRO" and published the original observation of the "Bursae Mucosae" and on "lymphaties". The

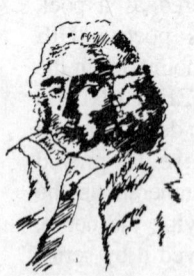
Monro primus
(1697-1767)

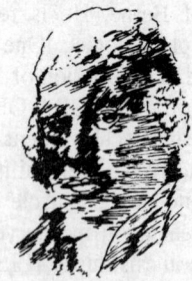
Monro secundus
(1723-1817)

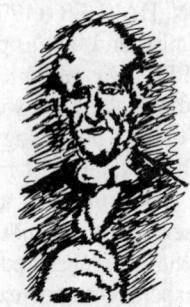
Monro tertius
(1773-1859)

Fig. 25 The Three Monros (1720-1846)

greatness of the secundus did not pass much to the next generation ALEXANDER MONRO TERTIUS (1773-1859).

During the early part of the 18th century Surgery was taught by the Professors of Anatomy. But gradually it was taught separately.

BENJAMIN BELL (1749-1806) was said as the first of Edinburgh Scientific Surgeon. He wrote a book "SYSTEM OF SURGERY".

Gradually different Chairs or professors were established for different subjects. They were mostly occupied by persons who had training from Leyden. In Edinburg tradition of Boerhaave and Leyden covered up the major part of the medical training.

ROBERT WHYTT

Among the great professors was ROBERT WHYTT (1714-66). He was the first to localise the seat of Reflex action in the spinal CORD, and to demonstrate that it was independent of the brain. His description of Tuberculous meningitis and of Diphtheria are a Medical classics.

To round up the rise and fame of Edinburgh Medicial centre it will not be befitting to mention certain names like SIR JOHN PRINGLE (1707-82), JAMES LIND (1716-1794), JOHN HUXMAN (1692-1768), SIR GEORGE RABKER (1722-1809).

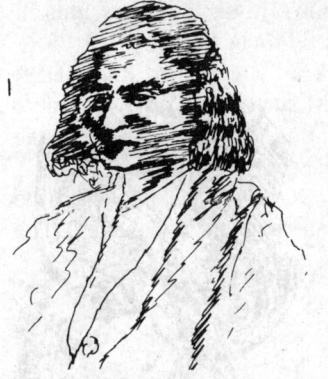
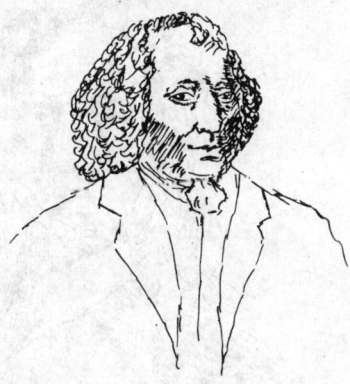

Fig. 26 SIR JOHN PRINGLE (1707-82)   Fig. 27 JOHN HUXHAM (1692-1768)

JOHN PRINGLE (1707-82): He was a M.D. of Leyden and was appointed as professor of Medical Philosophy. In 1742 he was appointed physician to the Earl of Stair, then in command of the British Army on the continent. At the battle of Dettingen in 1743, it was on Pringle's suggestion that negotiations and arrangements were made with French Commander that military hospitals on both sides should be considered as "SANCTURARIES" and should be protected mutually by both the sides.

This arrangements "TO PROTECT" rigidly led eventually to the development of RED CROSS.

In Oct. 1863 at the Geneva Conference an international arrangement was reached regarding the protection of the sick and wounded of the War casualities and those who attended them. In the following years the convention preassembled and resolutions were adopted to the declaration of a neutral status to all persons in attendance of the sick and wounded and the emblem of the RED CROSS was taken as their distinguishing mark. In 1752 Pringle published his observation on the "Diseases of the Army". Among his other works were a series of short papers on "Experiments upon Septic and Antiseptic substance" in which the word "ANTISEPTIC" was used for the first time.

About the same period there was another navy Surgeon "JAMES LIND" (1716-1794). His long service in the navy helped him to gain experience the influence of cold, damp and diets on the sailor. In 1753 he wrote a book on "TREATISE ON SCURVY", which was a classic literature in medicine.

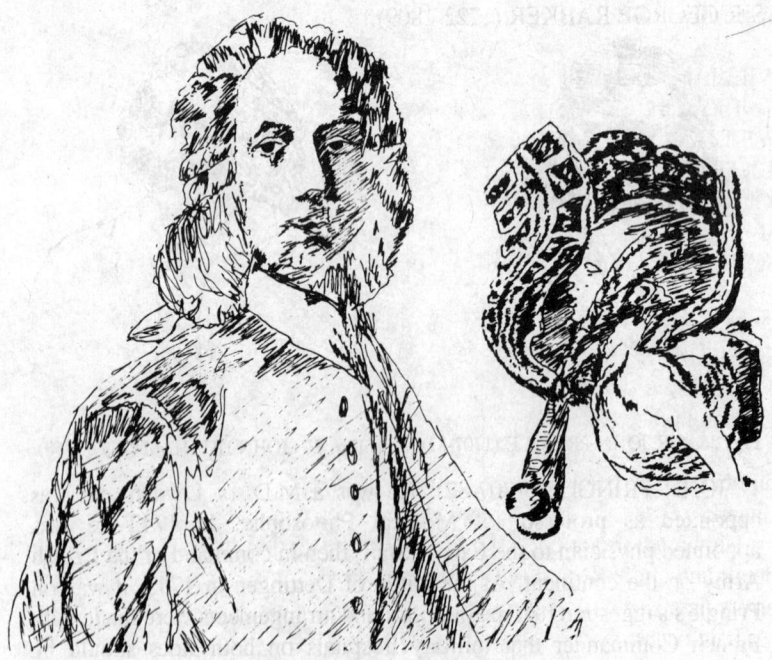

Fig. 28 WILLIAM SMELLIE (1697-1763)
Fig. 28.a Smellie's long Forcep, the blades bound with leather strips.

Lind was not the first man to suggest to use lemon or lime juice for scurvy. It was JOHN WOODALL, one of the queen Elizabeth's Surgeon (1569-1643), who served the East India company and JOHN HUXMAN (1692-1768) a well known Physician recommended the use of cider and vegetable diet as a means of preventing scurvy. The peculiar type of colic which was said as "Devenshire colic" studied by Huxman was proved by SIR GEORGE BAKER as a "LEAD COLIC".

In the later part of the eventful 18th century surgery was in the hand of Cheselden, Pott and John Hunter. In Medicine leaders were Radcliffe, Mead, Fothergill, Lettson, Withering, Baillie, Heberder and many others. The other branch which came up on a scientific basis was Obstetrics.

In the early days obstetrics was practised by the midwives only, gradually a change was brought by a type of specialists knowns as "MAN-MIDWIFE".

There were a number of persons who contributed in the field of obstetrics. Among them were a WILLIAM HARVEY, the first English man who wrote a paper on the subject (1651) and SIR RICHARD MANNINGHAM who laid a foundatin of "Lying-in" ward in obstertrics.

WILLIAM GIFFARD

There were some other persons who contributed in obstertrics. WILLIAM GIFFARD the first after Chamberlens to use 'EXTRACTOR or FORCEPS' (1726) and 'EDMUND CHAPMAN who illustrated and describe the forceps (1733). SIR FIELDING OULD of Ireland was famous for rendering help to establish "DUBLIN SCHOOL OF MIDWIFERY", a progress in the teaching of midiwifery.

In the British island the best man in the Midwifery was WILLIAM SMELLIE (1697-1763).

He studied in Glasgow and after a short training a Paris settled in London in the year 1739.

He was the leading obstetrician during his time and had large number of students. His large library was donated to the council of Lanark.

He wrote a book on "TREATISE OF MIDWIFERY" which gave a detail and clear account of the mechanism of labour an corrected many errors practised during the time.

It is occasionally said that SMELLIE was the inventor of Forcep, but it was not so.

He was one of the foremost persons to use forcep. There was a

Glimpses of History of Medicine

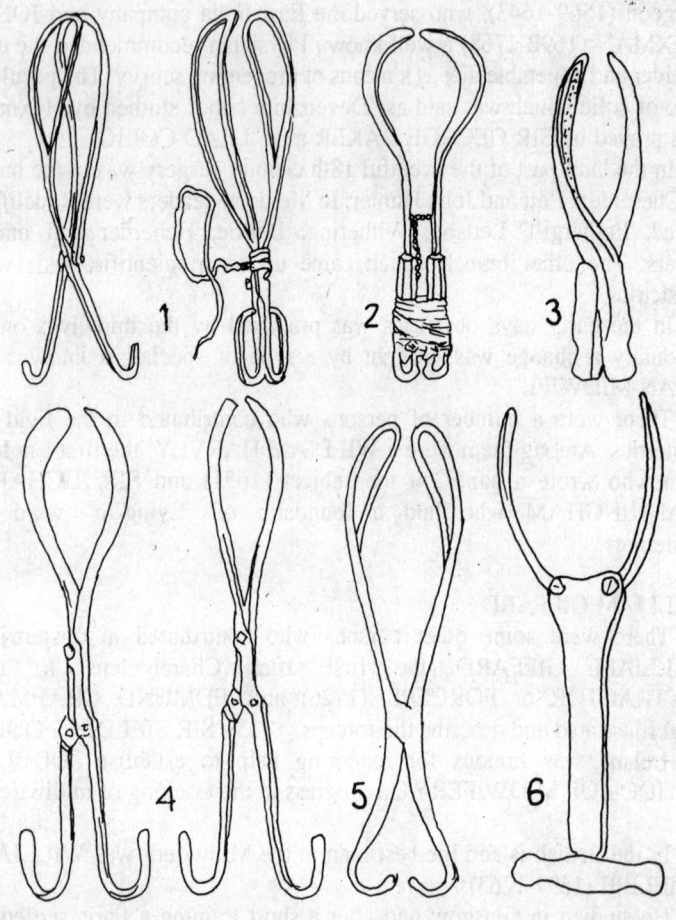

Fig. 29
1. Forcep invented by peter Chamberlen (the elder) about 1630 and retained as a family secret.
2. Palfyn's Forcep, two spoon with handles clamped together.
3. Smellie's short wooden forcep with English lock.
4. Dusees Forcep, the first attempt to articulate palfy's instrument by means of French lock.
5. Chapman's Forcep 1733; the blades united by a simple groove easily detachable.
6. Burton's Forcep 1751; Slender blades controlled by screw handle.

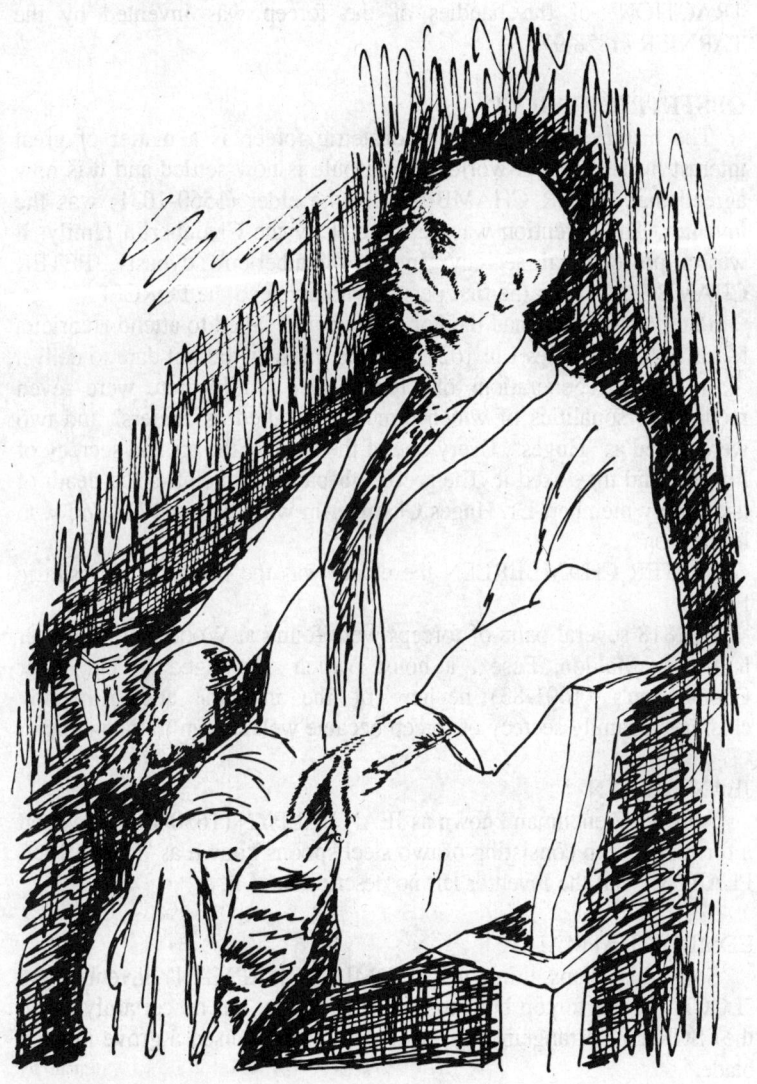

Fig. 53 Manuel Garcia in his hundredth year. Garcia was fifty years old when he invented the laryngoscope in 1855.

prejudice to use the forcep by the patients and practicing midwives, yet Smellie had the courage to go against prejudice.

Smellie at first employed WOODEN FORCEP, later on he had "METAL BLADES FORCEP" covered with LEATHER. The "AXIS TRACTION" of the handles of the forcep was invented by the TARNIER (1828-97).

OBSTETRIC FORCEP

The history of invention of obstetric forcep is a matter of great interest in the medical world. The dispute is now settled and it is now agreed that PETER CHAMBERLEN the elder (1560-1631) was the inventor. The invention was kept secret by the Chamberlin family. It was a professional secrecy. In the chamberlen's dynasty, PETER CHAMBERLIN was the first person who invented the FORCEP.

Peter Chamberlin had the honour of being called to attend Henrietta Maria wife of Charles I in 1628 after the midwife did not dare to deliver.

In the four generations of Chamberlin's family there were seven medical personalities of which three were called as "Peters" and two were called as "Huges". Every one of them knew the art and secrecy of Forceps and they used it. The secrecy became public after the death of last family member, Dr. Huges Chamberlin who died in 1728 and who left no son.

"PETER CHAMBERLEN the elder" was the inventor of obstetric Forcep.

In 1818 several pairs of forceps were found at Woodham Mortimer hall near Maldon, Essex, a house which belonged to Dr. Peter Chamberlen's (1601-83) nephew of the inventor and ultimately chamberlis family secrecy of forcep became well known to the public.

JEAN PALFYN

Another Frenchman known as JEAN PALFYN (1650-1730) devised a form of forcep consisting of two steel spoons known as "MAINS DE PLAFYN". But the inventor left no description of it.

EDMUD CHAPMAL

Some historians think that "EDMUD CHAPMAN" invented the "LOCK" in the forcep but possibly it is not so, but he certainly made the "SCREW" arrangements, the french idea and used a grove in each blade.

WILLIAM SMELLIE (1697-1763) invented the English Lock system and added flanges to the groves.

The pelvic curve seems to be independently introduced by Pugh probably.

The double curvature to the long forcep was introduced by WILLIAM SMELLIE.

William Smellie acquired a practice in Obstetrics and to whom William Hunter came as resident pupil in 1741. Smellie introduced the steel lock forcep in 1744 and the curved and double curved forcep during 1751-53. Smellie's "MIDWIFERY (1752)" was the first book to lay down safe rules for using forceps and for differentiating contracted from normal pelvis by actual measurement.

There are records that ANDRE LEVERT in 1747 showed his forcep with "La nouvelle courbourne" in Paris Academy.

In the early years of 18th century there were two leading personalities in Surgery William Chesel Den and Percivall Pott but they were superceded by their pupil JOHN HUNTER.

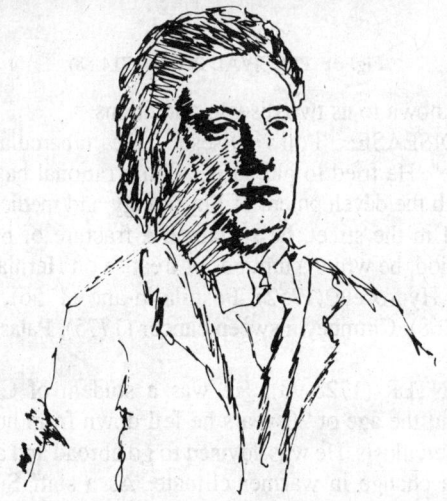

Fig. 30 WILLIAM CHESELDEN (1688-1752).

WILLIAM CHESELDEN (1688-1752): He was one of the famous surgeons of his time. He had the opportunity to attend SIR ISAC NEWTON and the Alexender Pope. He was the first man to perform Iridectomy and he had nice hand, for removing stones. "Fubham Bridge" a wooden structure spanning the Thames was built to his design in 1729.

PERCIVAL POTT (1714-88) : Another Contemporary of Cheslden was Percivall Pott. He was not only a good surgeon but had the inqusitiveness to find out some thing new.

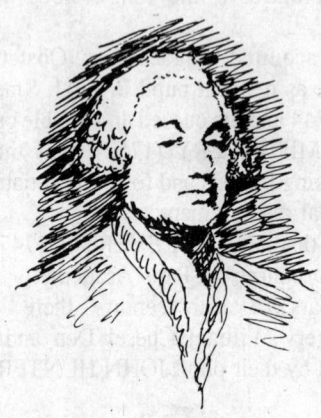

Fig. 31 PERCIVAL POTT (1714-88)

He is still known to us two disease conditions.

POTT'S DISEASE: "Pott's Disese"- the tubercular Spine and "Pott's fracture". He tried to put surgery on a rational basis keeping in conformity with the development of Physiology and medicine.

After a fall in the street, he sustained a fracture of bibula. During bed ridden period, be wrote a number of treatise on Hernia (1756) Head injury (1760), Hydrocele (1752), Fustula-in-ano (1756), Fracture and dislocation (1768), Chimney a sweep cancer (1775), Palasy from spinal carries (1779).

JOHN HUNTER (1728-93): He was a student of Cheselden and Pott. Near about the age of 20 years he fell down from horse back and developed Tuberculosis. He was advised to go abroad and as such joined the army for a change in warmer climate. As a staff Surgeon in the army, he spent four years in Belle Isle and Portugal. Prior to falling from horse back he was assisting his brother "WILLIAM".

Hunter was a man of composite character so his work was many sided. He collected about 13,000 specimens with the help of his students. He described the ramification of the olfactory nerve in the nose, the arterial supply of the gravid uterus and discovered the lacrimal ducts in man and many features of the lymphatic system. During this part of the century Surgery ceased to be regarded as a mere technical mode of treatment and began to take its place as a branch of scientific medicine, firmly grounded in physiology and pathology. His

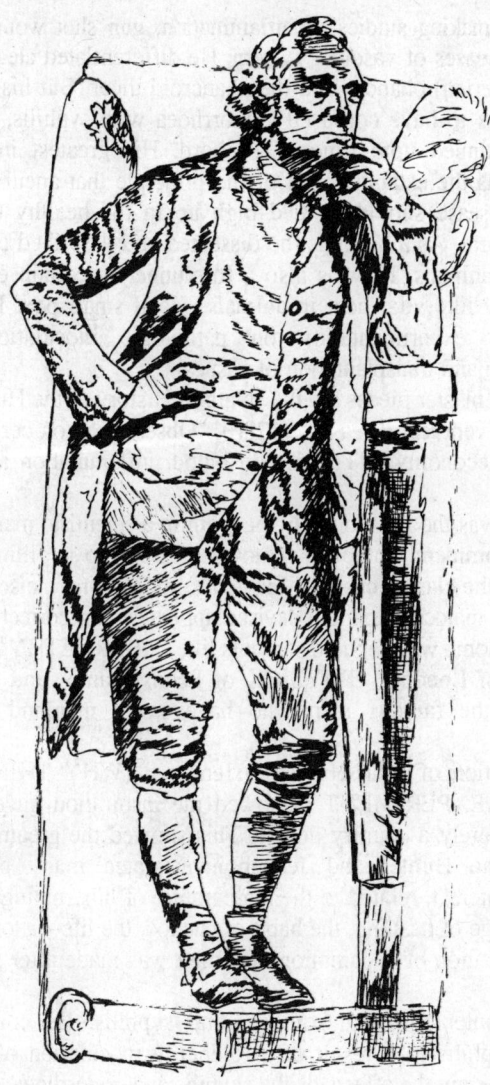

Fig. 32 Statue of John Hunter (The Museums, Oxford). (Courtesy of Professor William Stirling, Manchester, England.)

observation of the collateral capillary circulation led to his method of treating aneurysms.

He accidentally inoculated himself with lues and purposely delayed treatment in order to study the disease in his own system. As a surgical pathologist he described shock, phlebitis, pyemia and intersusception and epoch-making studies of inflammation, gun shot wounds, and the surgical diseases of vascular system. He differentiated clearly between hard (Hunterian) chancre and the chancroid ulcer. But his auto inoculation seems to have confused Gonorrhoea with syphilis, a confusion which continued upto time of Richord. His greatest innovation in Surgery was the establishment of the principle that aneurysms due to artificial disease should be tied high up in the healthy tissues by a single ligature. As a biologist he dissected and described 500 different species of animals. He was also a forerunner in certain experimental morphology like vital heat in animals, foetal small pox. He is also a pioneer in experimentation on pathologic inoculation and on regeneration and transplantation of tissues.

His four master pieces are the "Natural History of the Human Teeth" (1771), On venereal diseases" (1786), "Observation on certain parts of the animal economy". "Treatise on blood, inflammation and Gunshot wounds".

Hunter was the first to study the teeth in a scientific manner and the first to recommend complete removal of the pulp in filling them. He introduced the classes cuspids, bicuspids, molars and incisors, enlarged upon dental malocelusion and devised appliances for correcting them.

He had some well reputed students like "ABERNETHY". "ASTELY COOPER of London" "PHYSICK of Pennsylvania" and "EDWARD JENNER" the famous men who have saved mankind from great mysery.

A quotation of John Hunter to Jenner— (WHY THINK ? WHY NOT TRY EXPERIMENT") showed the inspiration gave to Jenner, who was merely a country doctor. This showed the greatness of John Hunter. John Hunter and Jenner investigated many problems of Scientific interest, related to the temperature of hibernating hedgehogs, the plummage of nestling, the habit of cuckoo, the life–history of else.

The invention of vaccination of Jenner was made after the death of Hunter.

John Hunter suffered from cerebral syphilis. He contracted the cerebral Syphilis as a result of a foolhardy inoculation of himself in order to ascertain the effects of the syphilis and gonorrhoea.

He died suddenly due to Angina when he was at a meeting of the Governor of St. George's Hospital.

Though he made no great discovery yet he was the originator of many discoveries.

WILLIAM HEWSON (1739-74): Hewson demonstrated the existence and function of lymph vessels and established that coagulation of blood is not because of solidification of the corpuscles but due to a

Glimpses of History of Medicine

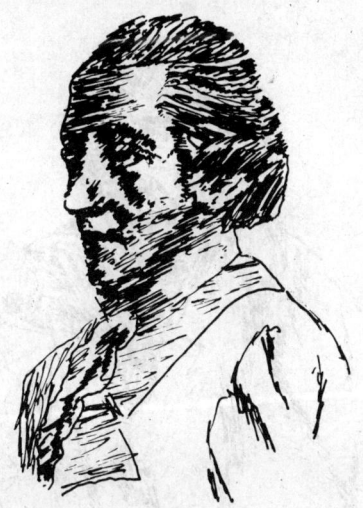

Fig. 33 WILLIAM HEWSON, F.R.S. (1739-74)

substance which he called it as "FOBROGEN.

JOHN ABERNETHY (1764-1831) was a pupil of John Hunter.

He was of opinion that all diseases which were not surgical or external were due to Digestive troubles and his favourite remedies were calomel and Blue pills.

Being a skillful and bold surgeon he was the first person to ligate the external iliac artery for Aneurysm SIR ASTELEY COOPER (1768-1841).

Cooper was a handsome and dignified in appearance and a careful operator.

Cooper's boldest operation was ligation of the aorta in case of an aneurysm. He was the first to amputate at the hip joint. He removed the Sebeceous syst from the head of king George VI.

His Royal Society memoir, on perforating the tympanic membrane for deafness resulting from obstruction of the Eustachian tube; gained him the Copley Medal in 1802 and his baronetey by a slight operation on George IV (1820).

His annual income was £ 15000. His servant "Charles" earmed £ 600 per annum from the patients by putting them out of was an another pupil of John Hunter.

During this period in Italy there was a distinguished surgeon known as ANTONIO SCARPA of Pavia (1747-1832). He was also a good Anatomist. His name is still remembered in many Anatomical

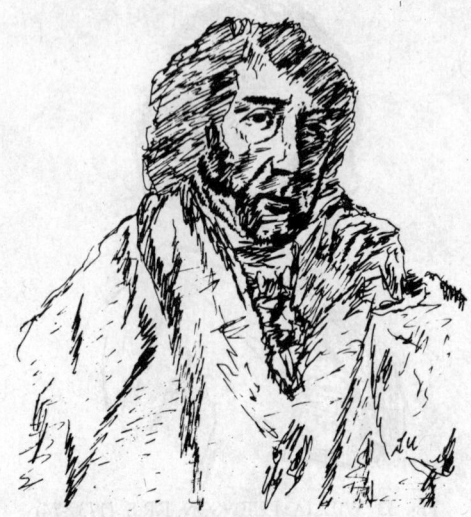

Fig. 34 ANTONIO SCARPA (1747-1832).

description. In anatomy, Scrapa is memorable for his discovery of membranous labyrinth, the nasopalative nerve, and the triangle of the high, which bears in his name. He was the first to regard arteriosclerosis as a lesion of the inner cost of the arteries and described the cubic-digital neuralgia (weir Mitchell's Causalgia) in 1832. He wrote important treatise on hernia and eye diseases and criginated the procedure of iridodialysis and made shoes for club-foot which is still the model for orthopedists. One of his Italian contemporary was DOMENICO COTUGNO of Napes (1736-1822) who discovered the CEREBRO-SPINAL and LABYRINTINE fluid and gave a presentive theory of hearing. He also wrote a famous article on sciatica.

During this period a name—ANTONIO VALSALVA of Bologna (1666-1723) was famous for his contribution in the field of Anatomy and Physiology of the ear.

In France the best surgeon was TEAN LOUIS PETIT. He was famous for the first man to trephine mastoid and to invent screw tourniquet.

On the other side of the Gulf in Persia there were two surgeons known JOSEPH DESAULT (1744-95) who respectively devised a better technique of amputation and treating fracture.

During the 18th century every body felt the importance of morbid Anatomy and Physiology (i.e., Pathology) for proper diagnosis and to know the etiology of the disease, which may be helpful.

Glimpses of History of Medicine 69

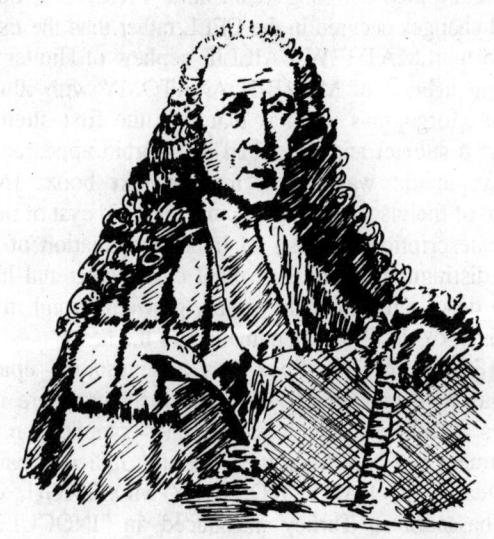

Fig. 35 GIOVANNI BATTISTA MORGAGNI (1682-1771).

The leader of the renaissance period of Pathology was GIOVANNI BATTISTA MORGAGNI (1682-1771). He studied under Valsalva at Bologna. A poet, an archaeologist and an anatomist of repute. He was engaged as a Professor of Anatomy at Padua at the age of twenty nine which he continued for fifty six years. He achieved fame for his ability to corelate Anatomy with Pathology with clinical medicine. He practised to make Postmortem and to corelate them with clinical dates. At the age of seventy two he published seven hundred case histories and their pathological findings. Among his contributions were the description of cirrhosis of Liver, Pneumonic consolidations of the lung, and different forms of tumour.

He first showed that Cerebral Abscess was the result of suppurative otitismedia. He gave the first description of cerebral gummata, diseases of cardiac valves, syphilitic ancurysm, tuburculosis of kidney, first recorded case of heart block and "Morgagnian cataract".

The knowledge of Pathology was further enriched by MARIE FRANCOIS XAVIER BICHAT (1771-1802) the pupil and assistant to Desault in Paris. Bichat founded the science of HISTOLOGY. He studied the Pathological changes occurred in the tissue or the membrane of twentyone type (i.e. cellular, nervous, bony, fibrous, muscular etc.).

His views were published in the year 1800. He was of opinion that pathological changes occurred in the tissue rather than in the organ. This views continued for long years until VIRCHOW observed that pathological changes occured in the CELL rather than the tissue.

The third man MATHEW BAILLIE nephew of Hunter contributed by publishing a book of MORBID ANATOMY with illustrations. It differs from Morgagmi's work is that it is the first attempt to lived pathology as a subject and described the morbid appearances of each organ in systematic way as in modern text book. He discribed transposition of the viscera, hydrosalpinx, dermoid cyst of the ovary and an accurate description cirrhosis of liver, hepatination of the lung in pxeynibua, distinguished ordinary renal cyst from renal hydatids. He gave a nice description of endocarditis, gastricular and in the second edition of his book described Rheumatism of the heart.

In the 18th century smallpox was a devastating epidemic. The mortality was high and among the survivors there were many pock-marked faces and cases of blindness and other complication.

The treatment and prevention were not on a Judicious basis.

In the year 1717 LADY WORTLEY MONTAGU, wife of the British Ambassador in Turkey introduced an "INOCULATION" in England against smallpox. It was first tried successfully upon six condemned criminals in England. Afterwards many members of the Royal family were inoculated. This increased the popularity of the method.

The practice of inoculation was present in East. In China the powdered dried crust from a case of smallpox was used as a Snuff in the nose.

The method employed in England was to make a superficial incision in the arm and to draw through it a thread soaked in the fluid from a smallpox pustule. It produced a mild form of the disease locally and the patient was safeguarded from future infection.

The method was so popular that "INOCULATION HOUSES" were establised and one of most famous inoculator was THOMAS DIMSDALE (1712-1800) a quack physician of Hertford. He inoculated EMPRESS CATHERINE and his son of RUSSIA. She was inoculated at St. Petersburg. Such was his success that he was made Baron and a reward of £ 10,000 with a pension £ 500 was given to him. He inoculated almost two hundred people in Moscow and St. Petersburg. His method was to make a small incision or a mere scratch. Children were incised during sleep.

Anyway it was beneficial to individuals but did not check the spread of the disease or reduce the mortality.

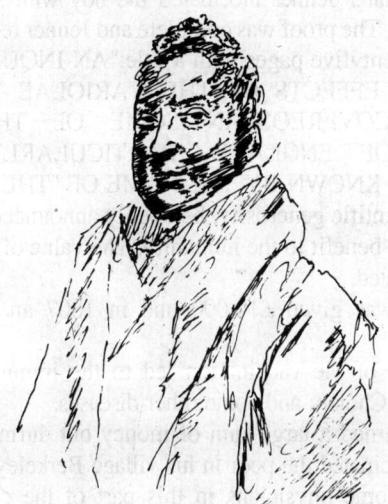

Fig. 36 EDWARD JENNER (1749-1823)

During this period there appeared a country practitioner named EDWARD JENNER (1749-1823), a beloved student of John Hunter. Jenner assisted Hunter in his research in Physiology and natural history. The love of nature and analytical observation of Jenner is shown in the writing of verses - "Address to Robin" "Signs of Rain".

He was the son of the vicar of Bearkley in Gloucestershire REY STEPHEN JENNER.

He practiced in his birth place and made the great discovery during his practice life.

The idea of vaccination was conveyed to Jenner by the remark of a dairymaid: "I cannot take smallpox for I have already had cowpox".

Cowpox was relatively a mild disease, transmitted from the cidder of the cow to the hand of the milkmaid or the milker. The infected person got a pustular eruption accompanied by a transient general Malaise.

Jenner considered the statement as true and thought this knowledge might be put to practical use.

For twenty years he thought on the problem and talked to his medical friends, who instead of encouraging, threatened him with expulsion from convivio-Medical Club, the local medical society.

At last on 14th May 1796 with courage he started the experiment and VACCINATED JAMES PHIPPS a boy of eight years with the pus from the hand of a dairymaid SARAH NELMES who had become infected with cowpox.

Eight weeks later Jenner inoculated the boy with smallpox and no disease appeared. The proof was complete and Jenner recorded his views in a book of seventyfive pages with a title:"AN INQUIRY INTO THE CAUSES AND EFFECTS OF THE VARIOLAE VACCINAE, A DISEASE DISCOVEREOS IN SOME OF THE WESTERN COUNTRIES OF ENGLAND, PARTICULARLY GLOCUESTERHIRE, AND KNOWN BY THE NAME OF "THE COWPOX".

With true scientific generosity, he openly announced his discoveries and made a great benefit to the humanity. The value of vaccination was proved and accepted.

In 1802 he was given £10,000 and in 1807 an another sum of money £ 20,000.

The principle of the vaccination led to the immunization of man against Typhoid, Cholera and some other diseases.

Though he earned a large sum of money but during the rest of his life he freely vaccinated the poor in his village Berkeley.

There were some physicians in this part of the century, who not only contributed in the field of medicine and materia medica but also public works for the benefit of the public more for the poor and a humane treatment for the insane the name of Dr. JOHN FOTHER GILL, JOHN HOWARD, WILLIAM TUKE, are worthy to mention.

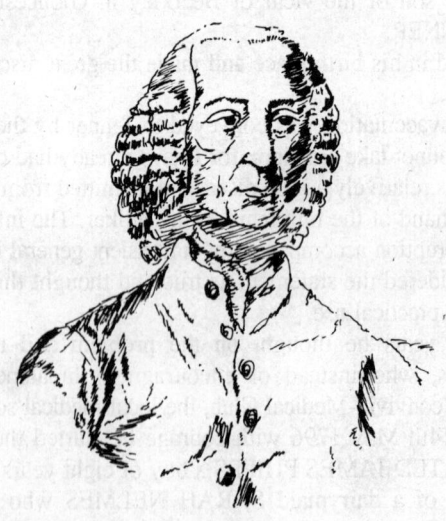

Fig. 37 JOHN FOTHERGILL (1712-80)

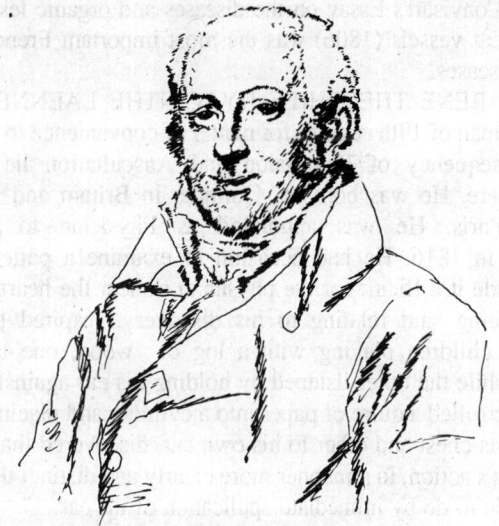

Fig. 38 Jean-Nicolas Corvisart (1755-1821)

CORVISART (1755-1821) of Paris, personal Physician and friend of Nepolean Bonaparte translated the book into French and accorded full credit to the discoverer.

It was possibly for the Auenbrugger to discover this, because he was

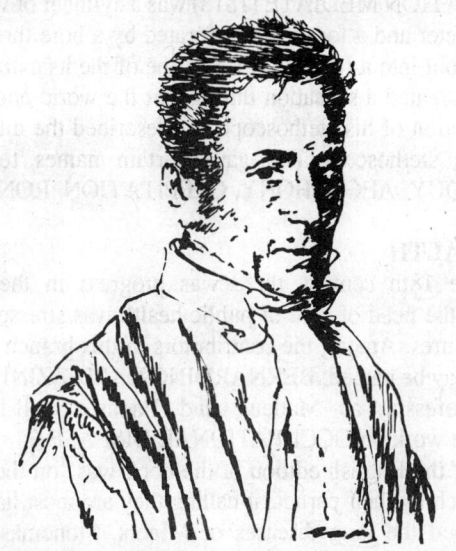

Fig. 39 Réné-théophile-Hyacinthe Laennec (1781-1826).

a musician. Convisart's Essay on the diseases and organic lesion of the heart and great vessels (1806) was the most important French treatise on cardiac diseases.

Although RENE THEOPHILE HYACINTHE LAENNEC (1781-1826) was a man of 19th century for matter of convenience to the reader to keep a sequency of Percussion and Auscultation he is being mentioned here. He was born at Quimper in Britain and ultimately settled in Paris. He was appointed as Physician to NEEKER HOSPITAL in 1816. He had occasion to examine a patient, whose stoutness made it difficult for the physician to hear the heart sound. A story was being said relating to his discovery. Inspired by having noticed two children playing with a log of wood, one tapping or scraping it while the other listened by holding his ear against the sawn end, Leennec rolled a quire of paper into a cylinder and placing one end on the patients chest and other to his own ear, discovered that he could hear the heart's action, in a manner more clearly and distinct than he had ever been able to do by immediate application of the ear.

Auscultation by direct application of the ear to the chest of the patient had been long known in medicine, even Hippocrates had described the "creaking as of leather which is audible in Pleurisy.

STETHOSCOPE

The Stethoscope described by Laennec in his book "TRAITE DE L'AUSCULTATION MEDIATE (1818) was a cylinder of wood one and a half in diameter and a foot long perforated by a bore three lines wide and hollowed out into a funnel shaped at one of the its extremities.

The work created a sensation throughout the world and he not only gave a description of his stethoscope but described the different sound heard by the stethoscope and gave certain names to them as - PECTORILOQUY, AEGOPHONY, CREPITATION, RONCHI.

PUBLIC HEALTH

During the 18th century there was progress in the community medicine and the need of care of public health was stressed by various hygienic measures. Among the contributors in this branch of medicine, few of them may be named: BERNARDINO RAMAZZINI (1633-1714) in 1700, Professor at Modeua and Padus, published a very comprehensive work on OCCUPATIONAL DISEASE.

The title of the English edition of the book was "on the Diseases of Artificers, which by their particular calling they are most liable to".

He described the lung diseases of Miners, Stonemasons, the eye diseases of blacksmith, gilders, lead poisoning of printers and potters.

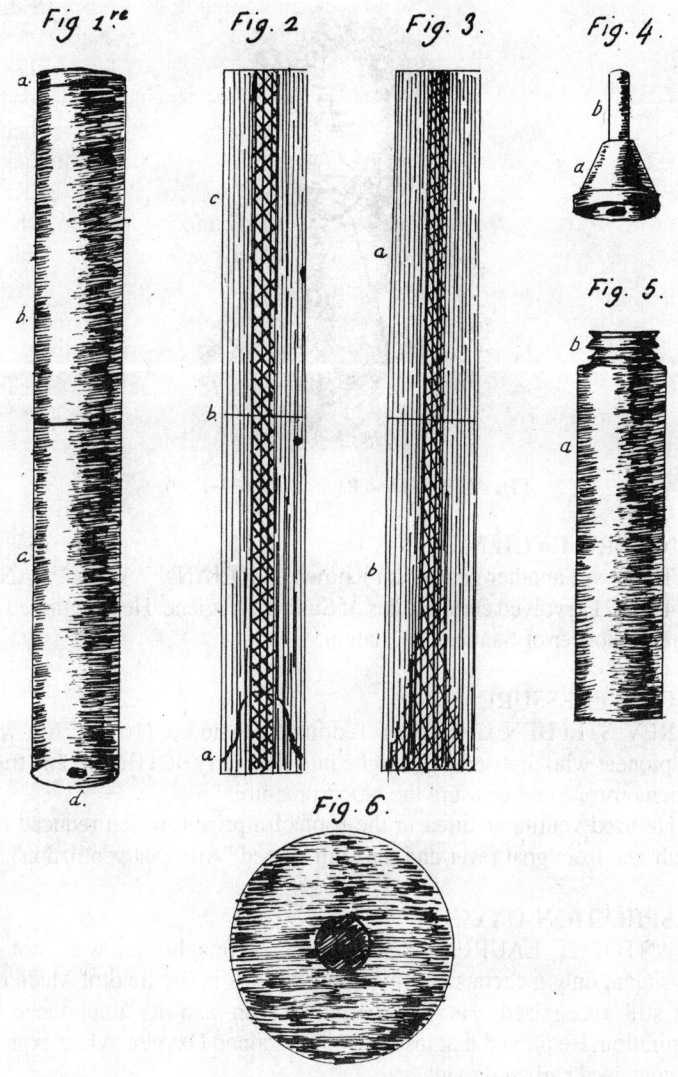

Fig. 40 Laennec's wooden stethoscope was designed as a more permanent substitute for his roll of paper. The Cylinder (Fig. 1) was made in two pieces, screwed together (Fig. 5) with a detachable funnel fitted into one end (Fig. 4). Figs. 2 and 3 show sections of the instrument with and without the funnel. While the end view (Fig. 6 natural size), illustrates the relative size of the bore.

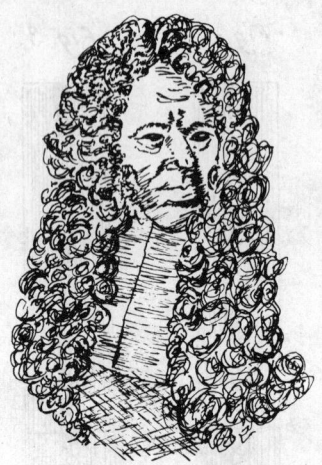

Fig. 41 Bernardino Ramazzini (1633-1714).

SANITARY HYGIENE

There was another gentleman Known as JOHANN PATER FRANK (1745-1821) evolved certain rules of Sanitary hygiene. He is regarded as a great pioneer of Sanitary legislation.

BLOOD PRESSURE

REV STEPHEN HALES of Teddington Middex (1677-1761) was the pioneer who inserted a glasstube into the artery of a Hoarse and tried to demonstrate and measure the blood pressure.

He used ventilator fitted in the roof of a prison, which reduced the death rate from goal fever and thus introduced "Artificial ventilation".

RESPIRATION OXYGEN

ANTOINE LAUREN ZAVOISIER: Though he was not a physician, only a chemist yet his contributions in the field of Medicine are still recognised. He discovered oxygen and its importance in respiration. He proved that inspired air contained Oxygen, while expired air contained carbon-dioxide.

He was a pioneer of hygiene, the first to demonstrate the chemical changes occurring during respiration and to show the necessity inhabitated buildings for a definite air space for each individual.

During the 18th century some unorthodox methods of healing were sponsored by medical men.

Prior to Lavoiser, there were two persons whose contribution could not be denied. They were JOSEPH BLACK and JOSEPH PRIESTLEY.

JOSEPH BLACK (1728-99): He was the Head of department at chemistry at Glasgow and later at Edinburgh. He showed that when mild line was burned into quik line. Previocusly it had been imagined that the line gained in weight, acquiring the mysterians substance "Phlogiston". Black disproved this idea noting also that the gas which he had discovered was a product of combustion and fermentation and that it was present in expired air. He named it "fixed air" van Halmant had called it "Gas sylvestre". Now it is familiar to us as carbon dioxide.

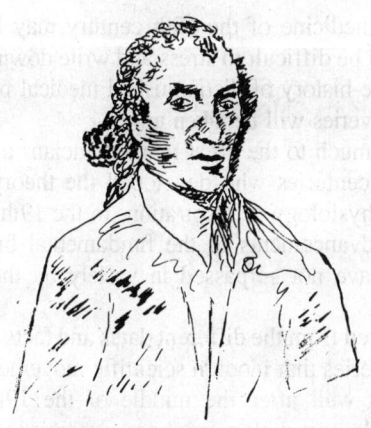

Fig. 42 Joseph Priestley (1733-1804).

JOSEPH PRIESTLEY (1733-1804): He was born at Leeds but died in America. He was accused in his home town because of his sympathy with French Republican and had to go to America for safety. He was a good Chemical research worker and he showed that growing plants were able to "restore" air which had been vitiated by product of combustion or of respiration or when it was treated with an acid, it lost in weight by yielding a gas and he actually prepared oxygen which he called "Dephlogistigated air" (1775).

Yet he did not completely solve the problem because he could not get rid himself of the mythical "Phlogiston" idea.

Demolishion of the phlogislon idea and the discovery of interchange of gases was possible because of gunices of Lavoisier.

MESMER

FRANZ ANTON MESMER (1734-1815): In the previous century

the cure of Scrofula by the "Royal Touch" was very popular.

Valentine Greatrakes an Iris man had achieved a great reputation for casting out evil spirits by laying on hand. Mesmer claimed that he could cure by touching. He practised HYPNOTISM by this means and ascertained that the secret of success lay in "animal Magnetism".

Originally he used Magnets, until he found that he could achieve similar results by the use of hands.

The credulity of mankind helped the Phaenology and Quackery to establish and few Charlatan exploited the people.

But with progress in all its branches of science including the medicine, made these charlatan to be more localised in their country-home.

The history of medicine of the 19th century may be so great and elaborate that it will be difficult to stress and write down each and every fact, as such the life-history of distinguished medical personalities and men of recent discoveries will be taken up.

Medicine owes much to the great mathematicians and physicists of the 17th and 18th centuries who developed the theory of vision and almost the whole physiology of respiration. In the 19th century though there were great advancements in the fundamental branches of pure Science yet they have not surpassed in variety by the works of any preceding age.

It may be observed from the different dates and facts (N.B.) and from the different discoveries that modern scientific movement did not attain its full stride until well after the middle of the 19th century. The medicine in the early part with a few good exceptions was only a part and parcel of the statutory or stationary thoughts and theory of the preceding ages.

N.B.— The physical principle of conservation of energy was demonstrated by Robert Mayer, a Physician of Heil bronn and James Prescot in 1842 and applied to the whole field of chemistry and physics by Helmholtz in 1847. The principle of Dissipation of Energy was first stated by Sadi Cannot in 1824 and developed by Clausius in 1850 and Lord Kelvin in 1852 and applied to all physical and chemical phenomena by Prof Willard Gibbs between 1872-78, the effect of Gibbs generalisation was so complete and far reaching that it made engineering, geology, biology, medicine to a new conception with the "States of substance" with the consequence to develop a new science—a Physical chemistry.

In physical or thermodynamic chemistry all changes of substance are treated as rigid consequences of laws of dynamics.

Kirchhoff and Bunsen in 1859 developed spectrum analysis. Faraday between 1821-54 and Maxwell in 1865 worked out on the theory of electricity and electromagnetism.

The Roentgen rays were discovered in 1895.

The curies isolated Radium Chloride in 1898. Thomas Young described Astigmatism in 1801, the wave theory of light in 1802 and surface tension theory of capillary in 1805, John Dalton stated the chemical law of multiple proportion in 1802, atomic theory in 1803.

William Hyde Wollaston investigated the pathological Chemistry of Calculi between 1797-1809. Darwin published his theory of origin of species (1859). As an inevitable consequence physics, chemistry, biology, medicine began to be studied as an objective science rather than human prepossessions.

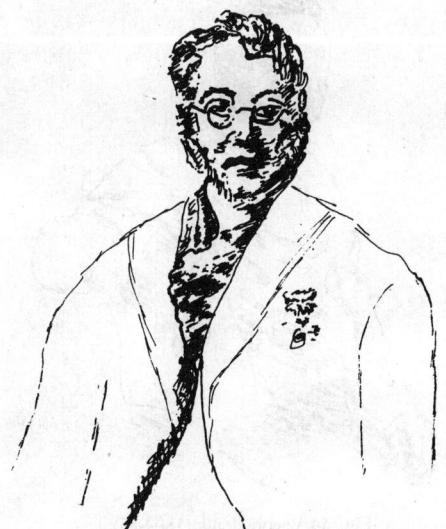

Fig. 43 Sir Charles Bell (1774-1842).

SIR CHARLES BELL (1774-1842): Since Harvey, Bell was one of the greatest discoverer in the early part of the 19th century. His contribution of the different functions of the Nervous system made him great. During his early part of life, he wrote a book for the artist. The book was known as "ON THE ANATOMY OF Expression"

In 1812 when he occupied the Chair of Anatomy in the Windmill School of Anatomy he dissected and observed the function of different nerves. His researches on the nerve made him to discover that there are two types of nerve—SENSORY and MOTOR, each subserving its own function. He opened the spine of an animal and "pricked the posterior filament of the nerve" and noted that no motion followed and then picked the Anterior filament and noted that immediate convulsion started. Thus the function of spinal nerve root was discovered. He discovered many other facts regarding the nerve i.e., LONG THORACIC or EXTERNAL RESPIRATORY NERVE OF BELL, which supplies the serratus Anterior a muscle which raises the ribs during respiration and the fascial nerve, paralysis of which develop BELL'S PARALYSIS.

He also proved that Surgical interference of the nerve.

All those discoveries, with case notes and drawing were published in a book "THE NERVOUS SYSTEM OF HUMAN BODY" a classic in medicine and possibly the first book on Neurology.

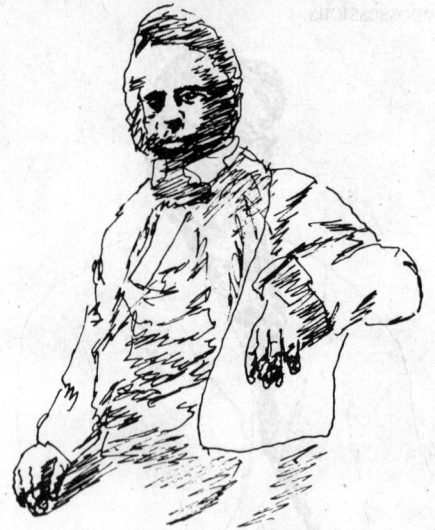

Fig. 44 Jacob Henle (1809-85).

HENLE

In this part of the century teaching of Anatomy gradually came up. throughout the world, in the continent DR. JACOB HENLE (1809-85) wanted to build up the knowledge of Anatomy from architectural standpoint and discovered the microscopic Anatomy. He wrote out a "HAND BOOK OF Systematic Anatomy" (3 Vol. 1866-71).

The handbook describes the macroscopic and microscopic structure of the entire body. Henle discovered the troubles of the kidney, the first to describe the epithelial coverings and lingings of the surface of the body, the muscular coats of the arteries, the minute Anatomy of the eye and various structures of the brain.

He was convinced that infectious and contagious diseases are caused by living organisms, which forecasted the present day conception of bacteriology.

JOSEF HYRTL (1801-94): A popular name in the history of Anatomy as an eminent anatomist and teacher.

He developed the technique of making "corrosion preparation" the blood vessels of an organ or a part being injected and then the alter tissue dissolved by the acid, so that all the vessels remained, clearly revealed.

Another famous name in the history of Anatomy:

HENRY GREY (1827-1861): He died at an early age from smallpox. Grey Anatomy descriptive and applied, is an immense popular book even today with thirty three editions. It was first published in 1858.

CARL ERNST VON BAER (1972-1876): A man who developed embryology and discovered the mammalian ovum in 1827.

While PAUL BROCA a surgeon of Paris (1824-80) who discovered the MOTOR SPEECH CENTRE and made out "LOCALISATION OF CEREBRAL CENTRE" of the brain and still remembered by us as "Broca's area".

Simultaneously with the Anatomy, the functional sphere i.e. PHYSIOLOGY came up very fast in this century.

The greatest exponents was JOHANNES MULLER (1801-58): Like John Hunter he was keenly interested in comparative anatomy but his greatest achievement was the publication of his HANDBUCH DER PHYSIOLOGIE DES MENSCHEN (1833-40), which is full of original observations and established physiology as a separate Science. He made discoveries in embroylogy (Mullerian Duct). He confirmed the findings of Sir Charles Bell regarding spinal root and its function.

He investigated the production of sound by vocal cords and he was the first to classify TUMOURS according to their microscopic appearance.

In his handbook he mentioned about the so-called Psychology and narrated the masterly account of mind.

Among his outstanding followers were HENLE, VIRCHOW as pathologist. HELMHOLIZ a master of physiology.

HERMANN VON HELMHOLTZ (1821-94): His paper on "CONSERVATION OF ENERGY" was published in Muller's "Archiv" brought him into prominence. Among other discoveries he elaborated the resonance theory of hearing and different papers to bridge the gap between the science of a costics and the art of music.

He established, by electrical means the rate of transmission of nerve impulses.

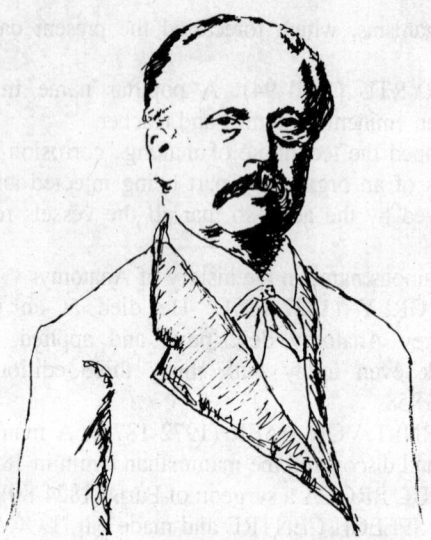

Fig. 45 Hermann von Helmholtz (1821-94).

He invented the OPOTHALMOSCOPE and had the opportunity to see the living HUMAN RETINA.

He made immense researches on mechanism of accommodation and problem of colour vision.

Another person THOMAS YOUNG, also made positive contribution on the problem of colour vision. This was confirmed by Helmholtz, and this theory was well known as "YOUNG-HELMHOLTZ" theory or colour vision.

Among many of his researches in the sense of hearing, the RESONANCE THEORY OF HEARING is still accepted to-day.

In 1871 Helmholtz was appointed as Professor of Physics and with the assistance of HEINRICH HERTZ in the matter of Electro-dynamics discovered the "HERTZIAN WAVES", which made modern wireless transmission possible.

EMIL DU BOIS REYMOND (1818-96) was the founders of Electrophysiological science and made numerous experiments on muscle nerve relations. His contemporaries in this field of work were AUGUSTUS WALLER who proved that the degenerative changes occured in the distal portion of a severed nerve and NERVE BLOCKING which is the foundation of one method of Local Anaesthesia of modern times.

Another contemporary in the field of Physiology was CARL LUDWIG (1816-95). He was regarded as the greatest teacher of Physiology who even lived during the present time. His contribution made much to advance the knowledge of Blood Pressure and of the

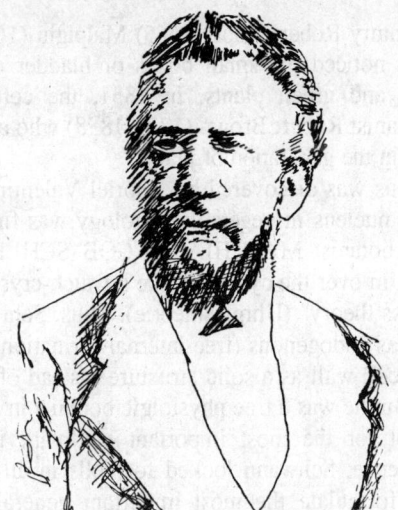

Fig. 46 Emil du Bois Reymond (1818-96)

functions of kidney.

MARSHALL HALL (1790-1857): He was a renowned British Physiolgist who openly denounced the prevalent practice of blood letting and unnecessary use of lancet. He remarked regarding lancet as a "a minute instrument of mighty mischief".

He studied hibernation, but his greatest achievement was the discovery of reflex action which originated from the observation that a headless neck moved when the skin was pricked.

The mutual relationship of the sensory and motor nerves and of the segments of the spinal cord from which they originated was noted by him.

Hall showed how reflex action occur, and also explained the act of coughing, the involuntary closure of the eyes when threatened, the breath of newborn child.

Another Physiologist WILLIAM SHARPEY (1802-80), who thought out that Physiology should not be an appendage of Anatomy and Physics. He made successful research on CILIARY ACTIVITY.

In the 19th century there were galaxy of masters; only a selected few are choosen in this chapter.

During the period the works of MATHIAS JACOB SCHLEIDEN (1804-81) and THEODOR SCHWAN (1810-82) and along with others are very important.

The development of the CELL THEORY, the most fundamental principles of modern biological science is keenly interrelated, was mostly the work of botanists.

In the 17th century Robert Hook (1665) Malpighi (1675) Nehemiah Grew (1682) had noticed the small boxes or bladder of air (cellular cavities) in cork and green plants. In 1831, the cell nucleus was discovered by botanist Robert Brown (1773-1858) who also discovered the role of pollen in the generation of plants

The cell nucleus was discovered by Gabriel Valentin in 1836. The significans of the nucleus in vegetable histology was first emphasised by the Hamburg botanist MATTHIAS JACOB SCHLEIDEN (1804-80). In the mean tim over the cytoblast like a watch-crystal over a watch, the "watchglass theory" (Uhrglastheorie). Thus, Schleiden regarded cell reproduction as endogenous (free internal formation) instead of by division, and the cell wall as a solid structure instead of a semipermeable membrane. But he was a true physiolgic botanist in tendency, with a lively contempt for the most important landmark in the modern history of the science. Schwann looked for cells in all the tissues he knew of and to formulate the most important generalization in the science of morphology, vix., the principle of structural similarity in animal and vegetable tissues: "There is one universal principle of development for the elementary parts of organisms, however different, and that principle is the formation of the cells." To Schleiden's concept of the cytoblast, Schwann added the "cytoblastema" or matrix of cell development analgous to the mother liquor from which crystals spring. This, as Virchow pointed out, was a tacit acceptance of "spontaneous generation," the very thing which Schwann afterward did so much to overthrow.

Theodor Schwann (1810-82), was the called to the of anatomy and at Liege.

A discovered the sheath of the axiscylinder of nerves, which goes by his name (1838), and the striped muscle in the upper part of the esophagus (1837). His inaugural dissertation (1834) showed that air is necessary for the development of the embryo; and, applying the same idea to the problem of spontaneous generation, he was able to prove, in 1836,[1] that putrefaction is produced by living bodies, which are themselves destroyed if the surrounding air be heated or vitiated. In 1837,[2] about the same time as Cagniard Latour, he discovered the organic nature of yeast, and showed that the yeast-plant causes fermentation which can be suppressed by heating the culture-medium and sterilizing the suroundign air by heat. As a physiologist, Schwann discovered pepsin in 1835,[3] showing its power to change nondiffusible

---

1. de Bary: Die Mycetozoen, 1859.
2. Schultze: Muller's Arch., Berl., 1861, 1-27.
3. Henle: Symbolae ad anatomiam villorum intestinalium imprimis eorum epithelii et vasorum lacteorum, Berlin, 1837.

albumens into peptones; and, in 1841,[4] demonstrated, by means of an artificial biliary fistula in a dog, that bile is absolutely essential to digestion. He was the first to investigate the laws of muscular contraction by physical and mathematical methods, in his classic experiment, demonstrating that the tension of a contracting muscle varies with its length (1835).

Thus the cell gradually came to be recognized as the structural and physiological unit in all living organisms, whether animals or plants, simple or complex, embryonic or adult, healthy or diseased, while, in our own time, the cell-nucleus is regarded as the chemical "centre of oxidation," the chromosome as the transmitter of inherited characters and the determinant of sex.

It was in this way that anatomic studies came to be more and more histologic or microscopic, and the "seats and causes" of disease itself to be referred to the cellular elements in the body and the unicellular organisms which may attack them.

The importance of the cell theory is immediately sensed in the work of Jacob Henle (1809-85), the greatest German histologist of his time and one of the greatest anatomists of all time. Born of Jewish parents at Furth, near Nuremberg, Henle was one of Johannes Muller's favourite pupils, one of his prosectors at Berlin, and later prosectors at Berlin, and later professor of anatomy at Zurich (1840), Heidelberg (1844), and Gottingen (1852-85). Henle did many important things for medical science. In his classic researches of 1836-1837 he was the founder of modern knowledge of the epithelial tissues of the body.

He first described the epithelia of the skin and intestines, defined columnar and ciliated epithelium, and pointed out that this tissue constitutes the true lining membrane of all free surfaces of the body and the inner lining of its tubes and cavities. In 1840, he demonstrated the presence of smooth muscle in the middle (endothelial) coat of the smaller arteries, a discovery which was the starting point of the present physiological theory of the vasomotor mechanism. He also discovered the external sphincter (striated muscle) of the bladder, the central chylous vessels, the internal root-sheath of the hair, the Henle tubules in the kidney (1862) and gave the first accurate accent of the bistology of carvea and morphology and development of Larynx.

In the century there appeared a number of physicinans whose names became attached to various diseases and symptoms. Among them the renowned one is RICHARD BRIGHT (1789-1858).

---

4. In his "Allgemeine Anatomie," Lepizig, 1841, p. 510, 690.
5. Contained in his "Handbuch der systematischen Anatomie4" 1862, ii, 300-305.

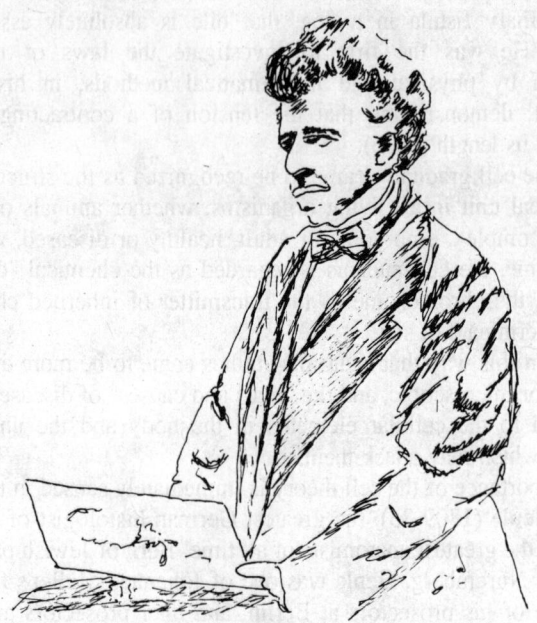

Fig. 47 Richard Bright (1789-1858)

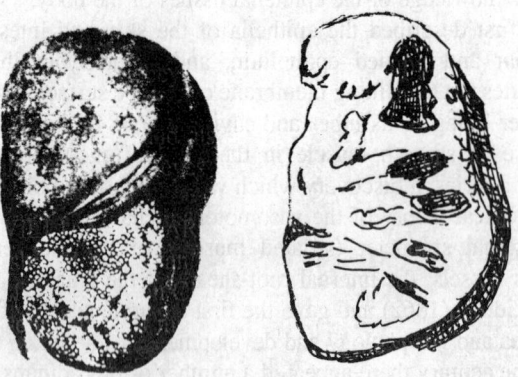

Fig. 47.a The kidneys of John King, a sailor who died of nephritis in Guy's Hospital. It was the study of this and other cases which led Bright to associate dropsy with disease of the kidney. The illustration is from Bright's Reports of Medical Cases, 1827.

He was not only a man of medicine but he has some original contribution in Botany, Zoology and Geology also.

BRIGHT was the first to point out that dropsy with albuminous unine was the result of kideny diseases. His observations appeared in the first volume of his well known "Reports of Medical cases selected with a view to illustrating the symptoms and cure of Diseases by a Reference to to Morbid anatomy (1827)". In this twenty three cases of renal diseases with post-mortem reports of fatal cases were published. In 1842 two hospital wards were set aside for his renal cases.

He also made keen observation on other diseases namely Abdominal tumours, Jaundice and Glycosuria.

He died at the age of sixty nine from Aortic valvular disease. He had a good friendship with THOMAS ADDISON, a colleague of Guy's Hospital.

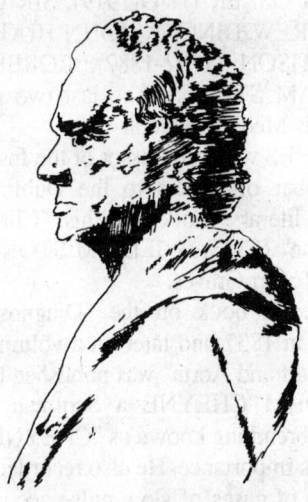

Fig. 48 Thomas Addison (1793-1860)

THOMAS ADDISON (1793-1860) also gave his name to disease. He graduated his M.D. from Edinburg, two years later after Bright. He was attached at Guy's Hospital; with Bright he wrote a textbook of Medicine which contained a good clinical account of "Inflammation of the Appendix vermiformis".

In 1849 Addison gave the first description of a remarkable form of Anaemia. He distinguished two separate maladies: one the anaemia which became generally known as "Pernicious" in which no organic lesion could be discovered; the other anaemia associated with brown skin with diseased Supra renal capsule. The later since then is called

"ADDISON DISEASE". During this century there was a leading London physician known as SIR WILLIAM WITHEY GULL (1816-90). He was very well known because of his certain remarkable comments, which is still worthy to remember.

They are - "NOT A TYPHOID FEVER BUT A TYPHOID MAN".

To a hysterical lady he remarked "THERE IS NOTHING REALLY WRONG; MRS X IS HERSELF MULTIPLIED BY FOUR".

Among his other aphorisms were "cannot is a word for the ideal and self satisfied; it is inadmissible in Science".

"Nursing is sometimes a trade, sometimes a profession, ought to be a religion".

In this part of the century many eminent physicians came in the field of medicine, who devoted much of their time in developing "CLINICAL MEDICINE" among them, the persons worthy to name are SIR WILLIAM OSLER (1849-1919), SIR CLIFFORD ALLBUT (1836-1925), ANDREW DINCAN, JOHN HUGHES BENNETT, SIR ROBERT CHRISTISON (1797-1882), ROBERT GRAVES (1796-1853) and WILLIAM STOKES. The last two persons were eminent physicians of the Iris Medical School.

ROBERT CRAVES was a professor of the Institute of Medicine and contributed a number of papers to the Dublin Journal of Medical Science but chief literary work was his "Clinical Lectures on the Practice of Medicine" (1843). WILLIAM STOKES (1804-78) was the life-long friend of Robert Graves.

Stokes published a book on the "Diagnosis and Treatment of Diseases of Chest" in 1837 and later on a voluminous literary work in "Diseases of the Heart and Aorta" was published by him.

Along with JOHM CHEYNE a Scotman practising in Dublin described a type of breathing known as "CHEYNE-STOKE" respiration and noted its serious importance. He also recorded along with ROBERT ADAMS a number of cases of slow pulse accompanied by syncopial attacks the "Stoke-Adams" Syndrome. During this period a life–saving surgical procedure called as "TRACHEOTOMY" was introduced by a French clinician PIERRE BRETONNEAU (1771-1862) who described Diptheria. Another important Surgical procedure was introduced by ARMAND TROUSSEAU (1801-67) to aspirate the pleural cavity. This procedure was improved by his pupil George Dieulafoy.

Throughout Europe there were many leading clinicians, who were contributors much or less in the field of medicine.

In Vienna there was JOSEF SKODA (1805-81): He devoted much of his time in chest diseases. He was conversant with the musical pitch which made him to contribute on Auscultation and Percussian.

In Germany CARL WUNDERLINCH (1815-77): He considered the Fever a disease left it a symptom. During this period another famous German clinician FRIEDRISH THEODOR VON FRERICH (1819-85) showed his great interest in Biochemical aspect of medicine and contributed original observations dealing with digestion, diseases of liver and diabetes. It was he who discovered LEUCIN and TRYSIN in the urine and acute yellow atrophy of the Liver. Sanatorium treatment in Tuberculosis was advocated by a Berlin physician EERNST VON ZEYDEN (1832-1910).

Similarly the man who first described progressive Bulber paralysis and diabetic coma and facts with disorders of speech and made pioneer attempts in oesophago-scopy and Gastroscopy was ADOLF KUSSMAUL (1822-1902).

The trend towards SPECIALISATION in clinical medicine came up gradually in this later part of the century in different continents and subcontinents.

Some Physicians tried to think diseases in relation to Biometeorological condition.

DANIEL DRAKE (1785-1852): An American medical man considered fever and other prevalent diseases according to Geographical predominancy, climate, diet, occupations.

There appeared brilliant pioneers in the field of GYNAECOLOGY-SURGEY namely EPHRAIM Mc DOWELL (1771-1830) and JAMES

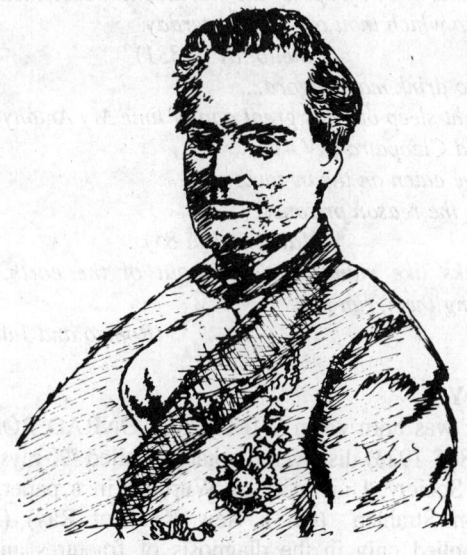

Fig. 49 James Marion Sims (1813-83)

MARION SIMS (1813-1883). Dowell performed OVARIOTOMY, a bold venture in those days when the knowledge of antiseptics or anaesthetics were not known to us.

SIMS became famous for operative treatment of VESICO-VAGINAL FISTULA.

The discovery of anaesthesia was a real addition in the field of Surgery. Painless surgery was a boon to the surgeons; still now no one is sure, who has really discovered the anaesthesia.

The network of the discovery started in America.

In the early days various drugs like opium, Mandragora and Cannabis Indica were used to relieve pain and to make the patient unconscious during surgical operation. Mandragora or Mandrake, one of the most ancient herbal remedies was used as an ingredient of the so-called Anaesthetic sponge. This plant is still found in the Mediterranean area. It has two varieties Male and Female.

As for its use in medicine, Dioscorides (First century A.D.) writes in his herbale that "the wine of the bark of the root" is to be given "to such as shall be cut or cauterised", and he notes that "they do not apprehend the pain because they are overborne with dead sleep". This is probably the earliest reference to surgical anaesthesia. Mandrake was also regarded as a cure for sterility. Shakespeare refers repeatedly to Mandragora and its effect as following quotations show:

Not poppy, Nor mandragora,

Nor all the drowsy syrups of the world, shall ever medicine thou to that sweet slup which thou ow'- dst yesterday.

(Othello, III iii 331)

gives me to drink mandragora....

That I might sleep out this great gap of time My Antony is away.

Antony and Cleopatra (I.V.4)

Or have we eaten on the in same root

That takes the reason prisoner?

(Macbeth, l iii 85)

And shrieks like mandrakes' torn out of the earth. That living mortals hearing them, run mad.

(Romeo and Juliet, Iv iii 47.)

RADIOLOGY

Radiology was born when WILLELM CONRAD ROENTGEN of Wurzburg (1845-1923) discovered what he called "X-rays" in 1986, at the Physical Society, University of Wurbug, in a paper, "Uber eine neue Art von Strahlen" (On a New Kind of Ray) (Plate LXX). Originally applied only in the diagnosis of fractures and of foreign bodies, the scope of the rays was soon extended to the recognition of calculu. The use of bismuth and later, barium, in the gastro-intestinal tract, and of various radioopaque drugs which are excreted through the biliary and urinary tracts, further increased the usefulness of X-rays. Still later.

Radiogram of the hand of Professor Kolliker, taken by Professor Roentgen when he read his paper announcing the discovery of "A New Kind of Ray" medhod was applied in the diagnosis of lesions of the brain and of the lungs. The Nobel Prize was awarded to Roentgen in 1901. Unfortunately the Roentgen rays were in use for some years before their harmful effects, in producing cancer of the skin in the operators, were recognized, and many an X-ray matrur to science met his death owing to lack of that adequate protection which is now universally adopted.

The therapeutic value of X-rays in skin diseases was early recognized, and lately deep X-ray therapy has been largely applied in malignant disease.

NIELS RYBERO FINSEN (1860-1904) deserves mention, as the recognised the effect of ultra-violet light upon the skin and its of modern ligttherapy in the Finsen Institute of Copenhagen.

Another notable discovery, that of radium in 1898, by the Curies (PRIRE CURIE (1859-1906), MARIE SKLODOWSKA CURIE (1867-1934) gave to the medicial a powerful agent whose final place in treatment of cancer is not yet ascertained. The bibliography of Madame Curie by her daughter, Eve Curie, fully deserves its wide popularity.

The list of special branches of medicine might be extended. Endocrinology, chemotherapy, nutrition, allergy, haematology, and other fresh sciences have afforded fresh fields for investigation and discovery. The results cannot yet be regarded as history, and therefore do not come within the scope of the present work.

The applications of Rontgenology to surgery and medicine were developed with amazing rapidity and in less than twenty years the new science was on a firmer footing than most. Rontgenography was immediately applied by the surgeon to the diagnosis and location of fractures, dislocations, foreign bodies, and embedded projectiles, by the denist to the teeth, by the physiologist to the elucidation of function, by the medico-legal expert to the detection of concealed objects and the diagnosis of death (Vaillant, 1907). An early pioneer was W.B. Cannon, who elucidated the movements of the stomach (1889) and intestines (1902). Further improvements in technique led to such novelties as pnemoperitoneum (Weber, 1915), ventriculography (Dandy, 1918) and cholecystography (Graham and Cole, 1923-24).

Rontgentherpy started with the discovery of the possibility of epilation in naevus pilosus and hypertichosis by Leopold Freund of Vienna (1896), favus (Freund, 1898), eczema (Hahn, 1898), superficial epithelioma (Stenbeck and Sjogren, 1899-1900) and alsopecia (Kienbock, 1900). The new period was ushered in by G. Holzknecht and Kienbock, who introduced disphragm (1902-3), which intensified the object by cutting out secondray rays, showed the injurious effect of the rays upon internal organs, notable azosperima (1903) and devised the leaden chamber for the protection of (103). Seen applied the x-rays to the treatment of leukemia (102-3) and Heineke noted their selective effect upon lymphatic organs (1903-4). Tubes of calcium glass (Grunmach,1905) and of lead glass (Wichmann, 1905) added to the comfort of the (1906) made for more distinct pictures. The observations on the effects of irradiation open the growth of young animals (Perhaps, 1903) in suppressing sweat (Buschke and Schmidt, 1905), on the leucoeytes (Aubertin and Beaujard, 1904), the testicle Hirschfeld, 1907) and in the production of cholin in the blood (Benjamin 1907) at Paris (1900). Berne (1902), and Milan (1904) and a Roentgen Society was founded in Berlin (1905). The pioneer work of Kienbock, Hoizknecht, Albers-Schoberg and Perthes was continued in France by Becle're (Paris), Bergonie (Bordeaux), Ledue (Nancy) and Bordier (Lyons), in England by Hall Edwards, Morton, and Sequeira, in America by Pusey, Senn, Coley, Williams, Baetjer, Beck, and Stelwagon. In 1904, Foveau de Courmelles began to treat uterine myomata by x-rays and during 1906-10 much was done by Holzknecht, Wetterer, Albers-Schonberg, and others in irradiation of uterine tumors and hemorrhage, while following Beclere's work on deep therapy in tuberculous lymphoma (1905), Holzknecht, Kienbock, Wetterer, Freund, Barjon, Beclere, and Rudis-Jicinsky did much for the treatment of surgical tuberculosis (bones and joints). The introduction of such new devices as the Coolidge tube (19131) and the Potter-Bucky diaphragm (1913-242) mark the beginning of a new period. Finsen's treatment of smallpox pustules by exclusion of ultraviolet light (1893) and of lupus by its concentration (1895), the invention of the mercury vapour lamps of Leo Arons (1896), Peter Cooper Hewitt (quartz lamp,1901), and Kromayer (1904), the discovery of radium by the Curies (1808), the applications of radium therapy of lupus (Danlos and Block 1901) and malignant tumors (Danysz, 1903) of ultraviolet light (1903) and Alpine sunlight (1910) to tuberculosis by Rollier, and to rickets by Kurt Huldschinsky (1918), along with the introduction of diathermy by Franz Nagelschmidt (1894) have extended the possibilities of phototherapy and Radio therapy to all manners of diseases and particularly in cancer.

PSYCHIATRY

Nothing is more impressive in medical history than the change of attitude towards mental disease which has then placed within the past hundred and fifty years.

It was in 1793 that the noble-minded PHILIPPE PINEL (1745-1826) boldly advised removal of the chains which restrained insane persons, at the Buicetre hospital of Paris 2. One had been chained for forty years, another for thirty-six years. Pinel affirmed that the mentally sick should not be treated as criminals. He introduced the idea of the mental hospital, in which mental disease would be treated like other forms of disease, and in which case-histories would be recorded and scientific such reforms during the yers of Revolution, and it is recorded that he was attacked by a mob, who accused him of harbouring that he was attacked by a mob, who accused him of harbouring refugees, and was liberated.

The new outlook upon "insanity" and "madness" was but slowly adopted, and even in 1830 JOHN CONOLLY (1794-1886), physician to Hanwell Asylum, was conducting an energetic campaign in favour of non-restraint. It became a subject of heated argument in all circles of society. While Pinel was still at work in Paris in 1792, William Tuke, a Quaker philanthropist, who was not a medical man, formed the Retreat at York, an institution designed to mitigate the unhappy fate of mental patients. Here there was no restraint and no chains, and the success of the enterprise did much to alter public opinion, and to hasten the adoption of humane treatment. Before the attempt of humane treatment of the insane, PHILIPPE PINEL (1745-1826) on 24th May 1798 struck of the chains of 49 insane patients at Bieetre with the consent of the National Assembly William Tuke's great-grandson, before Kraepelius, JOHN CONDLLY (1885) also advocated open door method (without mechanical restraints) in the treatment of insane.

Another person WILHELM GRIESINGER (1817-1887) of Stuttgart wrote a famous treatise on "Pathology and Therapy of Psychic disorders" and did with much of the mysticism of the past and gave clear and unmistakable chemical pictures based upon, rational psychological analysis aimed to connect the subject with pathology, anatomy, Psychiatrical clinic. Danien Hack Tuke (1827-95), DANTEL HACK TUKE (1895), studied medicine and became a psychiatrist. He also was associated with the York Retreat1 (p. 249). An enlightened and scholarly man, he did much to raise the status of his specially in Britain and America. His many contributions to the subject were published in the Journal of Mental Science, of which he was editor. Another editor of this journal, and also a Yorkshireman, was HENRY MAUDLEY

(1835-1918), who practised in London.[2] He wrote extensively on the mutual insanity with crime.

Sir THOMAS SMITH CLOUSTON (1840-1915) of Edinburg, was an excellent teacher of psychiatry. His textbook of Mental Diseases was widely used, while his work on The Hygiene of Mind is full of salutary advice, and foreshadowed the present-day vogue for popular expositions of psychology.

In Germany the leading exponent of psychiatry was EMIL KRAEPELIN (1855-1926), most of whose work was done at Munich-3. His monumental textbook describes the two major groups of mental disease—the manic depressive psychoses and dementia praecox, the former usually curable, the later incurable. Kraepelin's system is no longer adopted, but he rendered good service by showing that mental disease follows a definite course, like many other diseases.

During Kraepelin period there were many famous men of psychology. The prominent among them were:

(1) CARL WERNICKE (1948-1905)

He was a professor at Berlin and contributed not only important facts of insanity but also of sensosy ophasia, alexia, agraphia, internal capsule etc.

(2) Kraepelin's Eugen Beluler (1857-), of Switzerland, has expanded of "schizophrenias" (1910) which imply many things not regarded by Kraepelin, in particular "autism," or the mental life of introverted or introspective people, who lead shut-in lives. Bleuler also described "relative idicoy" (1914).

(3) Adolf Meyer (1866-), of Switzerland, professor of psychiatry at the Johns Hopkins University (1910) has steered and maintained a middle course between behaviourism and introspection, basing his psychiatry upon "psychobiology," which makes no sharp division between physiologic and psychologic data, but envisages mental phenomena as "higher and more complicated (frontal lobe) integrations or sublimations of the instinctive processes originating in the brain-stem."

(4) Richard von Krafft-Ebing (1840-1902), of Mannheim, a pupil of Friedreich and Griesinger, professor at Strassburg (1872), Graz (1873), and Vienna (1889), wrote the best German work on forensic psychiatry (1875), also a treatise on psychiatry based upon clinical experience (1879), and is especially known for his Psychopathia sexualis (1886), which classifies and describes the various forms of sexual inversion and perversion, especially in their medic-legal relations. Theodor Ziehen (1872-), of Frankfurt, A. M., professor at Jena (1892), is remarkable for his work on physiological psychology

(1891-1898), morphology of the central nervous system (1892-1899), and the psychopathology of the children (1902-1917).

(5) Of the French psychiatrists, Jules Baillarger (1809-1890) investigated manic-depressive insanity as folied double forme (1853-1854) and cretinism (1873), and founded the Annee medico-psychologique (Paris, 1843), now edited by Henri Colin (1921). Paul Serieux (1864-) wrote on reasoned insanity (with Capgras, 1909). Rene Semelaigne (1855-) made valuable study of the Pinels and the Tukes (Alinenistes et philanthropes, 1912).

(6) Of English psychiatrists, Sir Thomas Smith Clouston (1835-1915), late editor of the Journal of Mental Science, wrote a volume of clinical lectures on mental diseases (1883); Henry Maudsley (1835-1918) was a prolific writer on psychological themes; Charles Arthur Mercier (1852-1919) was author of a text-book (1902), but his most valuable contributions are those on criminal responsibility (1905), conduct and its disorders (1911), crime and insanity (1911), and his historical studies of astrology (1914) and leper houses (1915); John Milne Bramwell (1852-) has written much on hypnotism; Sir Frederick Walker Mott (1959-1926), editor of Archives of Neurology, was author of the Croonian lectures on the degeneration of the neuron (1900). L. S. Forbes Winslow (1844-1913) wrote treatises dealing with the legal (1874) and picturesque aspects of lunacy (1898-1912), and entertaining memoirs (1910).

(7) Hugh Crichton Miller (1877-) has written interestingly on hypnotism. Mention should be made of the Italians, Sante de Sanctis (dementia praecosissima, 1906), Giovanni, Mingazzini (encephalitis lethargica, 1921), Eugenio Tanzi (1904), and Leonardo Bianchi (1905), whose psychiatric treatises have been Englished; of the Russians, Ivan Pavlovich Merzheyevski (1838-1908), Nikilai Nikolaievich Bazhanoff (1857-), Ivan Alexandrovich Sikorski (1845), notable for his work on physiognomy of the insane (1887-93), Sergiei Sergievich Korsakoff (1853-1900), who described polyneuritic insanity (1887) and wrote a text-book (1893), and Vladimir Michailovich Bechtereff (1857-1927), author of a classification on insanity (1891), a neurological treatise (1894-1899), and psychiatric lectures (1908); and of the Americans, Edward Charles, Spitzka (1883), Henry J. Berkley (1900), Stewart Paton (1905), and William A. White (1909). As superintendent of the Government Hospital for the Insane (1903), editor of the Psychoanalytic Review, and author of a treatise on mental mechanisms (1911) White has done much for recent psychiatry. With Smith Ely Jelliffe (1866-), of New York, editor and translator of many things of historic interest and value, White collaborated in a treatise on diseases

of the nervous system (1915), presenting most advanced views of the nervous and psychic mechanisms as transformations of energy. Henry Mills Hurd (1843-1927), professor of psychiatry (1889-1911), was editor of The Institutional Care of the Insane in the United States and Canada (1916), which contains his valuable history of American psychiatry.

New methods of psychopathological investigation were introduced by Robert Sommer (1899). Psycho-analysis was introduced by Sigmund Freud had C. G. Jung (1893-1909). General paralysis of the insane was described by John Haslam (1798) and Calmeil (1826), moral insanity by James Cowles Prichard (1835), circular insanity by Jean-Pierre Falret (1854); hebephrenia by Karl Kahlbaum (1863) and Hecker (1871), katatonia by K. Kahlbaum (1874), psychasthenia by Pierre Janet (1903), presenile dementia, with plaques in the brain (1911) by Alois Alzheimer (1864-1915). A valuable contribution is that of Broussais (De l'irritation et de la folie, 1828). who like Stahl, was at his best in the psychic field (Zillboorg). Paul Briquet (1796-1881) published a monumental treatise on hysteria (1859). Alcoholic paraplegia, already noted by James Jackson (1822) and Sir Samuel Wilks (1868), was described as a polyneuritic psychosis by Sergiei Korsakoff (1887). Heinrich Laehr (1820-1950), editor of the Allgemeine Zeitschrift fur Psychiatrie (1858-), made valuable directories of the insane asylums of the Germanic countries (1852-1882), an unrivaled bibliography of the literature of psychiatry, neurology, and psychology from 1459 to 1799 (1900), and a calender of psychiatry (1885) containing, day be day, all the important events connected with the history of the subject, including the martyrology of physicians and asylum attendants killed by the homicidal insane. Otto Monkemoller has written well on the history of psychiatry (1903-1910)

Meanwhile, in 1885 to be precise, there was working in Charcot's clinic in Paris a young man who was destined to revolutionize psychiatry, and indeed to change the outlook to revolutionize psychiatry, and indeed to change the outlook in the whole field of medicine. Darwin and Husley, the outlook in the whole field of medicine. Darwin and Huxley, by viewing man from a zoological standpoint, had profoundly influenced the current of medical thought. In like manner Freud, by his discovery of the unconscious mind, altered the trend of medicine, and gave a salutary check to the materialistic tendencies of the age of specialism. SIGMUND FREUD (1856-1939), who revolutionized the entire field of psychology, lived most of his life in Vienna.[4] In his autobiography he tells us that in 1889 he realized that "there could be powerful mental processes which nevertheless remained hidden from the consciousness of men."[5] From this idea evolved his system of "psycho-analysis" and found that he could dispense with hypnotism, which he had been employing. Freud's principles, now so familiar, were only slowy adopted, and at first he was severely criticized on account of his preoccupation with sex psychology. Despite the opposition, his discovery of the unconscious mind was more important than any other in the whole history of mental disorders. He showed, moreover, that there was no clear borderline between normal and abnormal psychology, and his ideas have assumed importance in almost every field of human activity.

Freud lived long enough to see his views widely accepted, although the end of his life was clouded, and he died in London as a refugee. The importance of the Freudian revolution is not yet fully realized. To-day, medical psychology is permeating all branches of medicine, and it may prove to be the activating factor of a new year in medical science.

Of recent years there has been an amazing increase in the literature of psychology, normal, morbid and comparative, including such related subjects as pedagogies, psychoanalysis, psychotherapy, epistemology, the scientific aspects of evidence and the relation of everyday thinking to border-line insanity. Psychology, defined by Jastrow as "a colonial outpost of philosophy or, heater, a protectorate of physiology" in its early phases, has steadily advanced through the physiological and psychological stages, to the comparative status, and is now an analogue of the general physiology of clande Bernard. Psycho-physies or quantitative psychology) as illustrated in the achievement of Wundt, Lotze, Fechner and Herbart, and of Mc Keen Cattell in America, tended to "Conceive sensations and Stimuli as abstraction even instrumenal realities like grammes on candle-powers or watts or ohms," and fell short of the profitable approach to the Living organism, which must necessarily be qualitative or genetic. Comparative Psychology turns mainly upon Loeb's theory of tropisms in the Lower forms (or the views of those who, like H.S. Jennings, oppose it) and the study of "behaviour" in the higher animals (Watson). The mental development of the newborn infant has been specially studied by Kussmaul and Preyer. Pedagogies and Juvenile psychology have been treated by Binet, Claparede, Stanley Hall, Seguin, Maria Montessori and others. Among the Leaders in morbid-psychology is Pierre Janet (1859), Professors at college de France, who developed the Theory of Psychologic automatism (1889), the relations between neuroses and fixed ideas (1902) described psychasthenia (1903), and made extensive investigations of the mental status of hysteric patients (1903-8), emphasizing, in particular, the sexual factor in hysteria, but with the sound view that the sexual inadequacy of the neurotic is a symptom and not a cause, and that much alleged morobid is the effect of bad domestic environment, the selfish hypocrisy of parents and such like, the selfish Alfred Binet (1857-1911) and Th. Simon introduced a series of graded tests for mental retardation by which it is possible to localize the developmental stauts of a patient's mind in relation to his age and the growth of his body (mental age), thus enabling school teachers or school inspectors to segregatge defective or "unusual" children. Another characteristic development is the exhaustive or intensive study of sexual psychology, with which modern writers, from scientific students like Krafft-Ebing and Haveloek Ellis, down writers, from scientific students like Krafft-Ebing and Havelock Ellis, down to insane men of letters like Krafft-Ebing and Havelock Ellis, down to insane men of letters like Nietzsche and Weinnger, have been vastly preoccupied. The atmosphere of the present time, its art, poetry, fiction, and drama, is saturated with sexualism. Poets like Goethe, Swinburne ,and Walt Whitman did much to dispel the ancient theological nightmare of the sinfulness of normal sexuality in men and women, and are forerunners of the scientific view that the instinct is an all-important part in normal human development, and has to be either recognized or reckoned with. Schopenhauer wrote on the subject with bitter and unsparing realism, and latterly women of such high repute as Rahel Varnhagen, Ellen Key, and Helen Putnam have considered the matter from a higher viewpoint, on account of its importance in connection with such problems as the proper hygiene and well being of growing children, the growth of prostitution and commercialized vice, the social enslavement of women in crowed communities, and other degradations of a purely industrial age. In Germany, several periodicals are devoted to the sexual instinct alone, and the problems of biological are devoted to the sexual instinct alone, and the problem of biological teaching of school-children in these matters is under consideration. On the pathological side, there is the question of sexual perversion and the crimes resulting from it, for which, in young, healthy frontier communities like the United States no special provisions have been necessary in criminal procedure until the crowded conditions of modern cities brought the unsavoury subject to the surface.1 Recent thinking has been revolutioned by the revelation of the part played by suppressed or represesed sexuality in the development of neurotic conditions, the special achievement of Sigmund Freud (1850-), of Freiberg in Moravia, a pupil of Charcot, and professor of neurology at Vienna. Charcot, as we have seen, threw the sexual theory of hysteria into disrepute. Janet introduced the eathartic treatment (questioning that hypnosis). Freud, in particular, interpreted the mechanism of hysterias the resultant of a psychic traumatism or nervous shock, of sexual nature in the first instance, leading to morbid brooding and a kind of mental involution. Freudians hold the sexual factor to be existent in normal people, but the way in which the individual reacts to the experience localizes the neurotic. The basic idea of Freud's subjective or dispositional psychology is that a large number of even ordinary mental processes come from hidden sources, unknown to the individual, whose tendency to fabricate reasons to justify the unsuspected reality is "rationalization" (Jones, 1908). Freud has also developed the theory of the psychic significance of dreams (Traumdeutung) and wittcisms as unintentional determinisms, infantile amnesia, auto-erotism (Ellis), unconscious memories, absent-minded actions, anxiety-neuroses, also various aspects of the "psychopathology of everyday life." He believes that there is a rigid determinism of psychical effects and that many complex mental processes never attain to consciousness and can be elicited only by a long process of "psychoanalysis," in developing which he was assisted by his pupil, C. G. Jung. Freud's first successful case, that of the patient "Dora," was of this kind. The correctness of his reasoning seems borne out by the successful treatment of hysteria through the disburdening of the mind or other appropriate psychotherapy. In his view, the basis of all sexual neuroses is the child's unconscious attachment to its parents, sometimes with hostility to the parent of the same sex. This "Edipus complex" White regards as the "family romance,"[1] symbolizing the struggle of the individual to attain to self-confidence and self-reliance by breaking away from dependence upon his parents. It is thus regarded as measure of the degree of infantilism in the neurotic. Freud's reasoning about the effect of the mind upon the body (psychogenesis), the ambivalence of emotions (Bleuler), the mental levels of the conscious, the subconscious and its censor (Hughlings Jackson), the opposition between day-dreaming (wish-fulfilment) and reality, transferences, fixations, repressions, sublimations and regressions, has exerted a profound, and, in its popular aspects, a very dubious effect upon modern thought. The real interest of Freud is his profound insight into the working of primitive mentality, or what Jelliffe calls "paleopsychology" (the historic past of the individual psyche). His school has occasioned abuses in medical practice and he himself has sometimes lapsed into extravagances of rationalization, which Jastrow wittily describes as giving "rich reasons for poor motives." In psychoanalysis, Freud has invented an instrument which can be exceedingly dangerous in intemperate, incompetent or unscrupulous hands. In America, his ideas have been followed by J. J. Putnam, A. A.

Brill, William A. White, and others, and such variants as Bleuler's theory of normal "autistic thinking" go to show the very partitions which sometimes divide sanity from insanity.

Among Freud's pupils, all of whom branched out for themselves, was Alfred Adler (1870), of Vienna, who stresses organic inferiority, sexual or other, as a prominent cause of neuroses (the inferiority complex, 1907). In this class of neurotics (Goethe's incomplete), the sexual or other inadequacy is set off by a constant subconscious effort to assert and attain superiority (Nictsche's "will to power"), the neurosis rooting in a constant overtaxing of bodily resources to compensate for the patient or latent inferiority. The strong deliberately choose plainness and simplicity. The neurotic, victimized by the "as if" tendency of Vahinger, acts on the assumption that he is strong, projects his own faults on to others, affects disdain, is fertile in reasons for failure, and combines a general faultfinding spirit with a self-imposed nimbus. This sound thesis Adler develops with great brilliancy, but lacks the lucid literary manner of Freud. Allied to this phase of constitutional psychology is Kretschmer's analysis of the manic-depressive and praecx (split personality) psychoses (1921). Janet's view of sexual inadequacy as a symptom rather than a cause of neuroses, is stressed in the writings of Wilhelm Stekel (1868-), of Vienna, which include an exhaustive analysis of the causes of impotence (1923) and an array of case histories which would have astounded Brantome. Both Adler and Stekel favour Janet's view that much of alleged morbid heredity is chargeable to unfavourable domestic environment, harsh parentage, family slavery, and so on. The effect of the modern wave of sexual emancipation has been to capitalize and commercialize the ideas of the Freudian school, with occasional untoward results in fiction, on the stage and in actuality.

In striking contrast with the psychogenic philosophy is the behaviourist (comparative) psychology, an analogue of general physiology, which makes a clean sweep of "mind" and its attributes as a mere concept in vacuo, interprets mentality in terms of reaction to environment, indeed maintains that from amoebea to man, the whole organism participates in thinking. Behaviourism was already implicit in the writings of William James, Stanley Hall, and others, but was specially developed by John Broadus Wastson (1978-). It derives immediately from which Watson applied to the nursery (1916). In Watson's treatises of 1914 and 1919, the centric idea of reaction to stimulus is developed with scientific exactitude which has own the approval of all and sundry. Where behaviourism fails is in the determined effort to apply the rationale of the conditioned salivary reflex to the higher reaches of consciousness and deliberate thought. What was applicable to the lower stages of behaviour becomes, in the words of Jastrow, "an acrobatic or verbalistic treatment, an ignoring of the realities, a juggling with formulae, such as stimulus and response, denatured of the very quality that gives them significance," in brief, "the grin without the cat," or "throwing out the baby with the bath." With reference to the two main trends which have dominated recent thought, Jastrow indulges the witticism that "psychology first lost its soul, and a change of mind." To see subconsciousness as virtually a sexual phenomenon, "a something not ourselves that makes for unrighteousness," is utterly to discourage the finer feelings and nuances of character. On the other hand, to envisage the human as a reliable feflex hound, registering salivary and movie emotions, is apt to make him seem, like Wilkie Collines' muscular Christians, "too unhealthily conscious of his unconscious healthiness," i. e., a dreadful bore. Here K. S. Lashley's important experiments on learning processes in rats (1912-26), as interpreted by Herrick (19261), may give us pause. Behaviourism has been most successful as comparative psychology, in elucidating the reflex life of animals, the infant, the anthropoid and the primitif. It is plain that in the higher animals, a function of the cerebrum (fore-brain) is to sublimate the instincts and affectivities radiating from the brain-stem and midbrain, that disorders of hunger (obesity), thirst (diabetes), sleep inter-brain (infundibular) functions, wherefore instinctive actions and sensing of personality have little to do with intelligence and intellect. A set-off to Freudian and behaviouristic reasoning is the Gestalt psychology of Kurt Koffka (1986-) and Wolfgang Kohler, which insists upon the psychic relativity of the laboratory animal, and the importance of the setting or background (Gestalt) as a configuration or constellation of factors. without which an object or happening has no significance whatever.

It will be most unwise if the name of Samuel Habnemann is not mentioned in this respect though he advocated different method of therapy yet he was also our of the person who strongly advocated humanly treatment of all mental discases including the insane. In the year in his book known as "Organon of Medicine" he said that mental diseases or insanity should not be taken as a separate one. They are the part and parcel of the total disorder or disharmony of the man as a whole. If the man is treated with special reference of the mental disorders; a better and judicial treatment may be reduced for a permanent cure.

As for its medicinal use, DIOSCORIDES during the first century A.D. made an reference of it anaesthetic properties.

In the town of Salerno, 35 miles south of Naples. the first organised Medical School called as "The School of Salerno" came up. Many eminents of Europe and other continents were trained in the school of Salerno. MICHAEL SCOT (1175 A.D.) was one of the famous persons got his training from this school. One of the Michael Scott's prescriptions cast an interesting light upon the early history of Anaesthesia. "Take opium, Mandragora and henbane equal parts, pound and mix them with water. When you want to saw or cut a man dip a rag in this and put it in his nostrils. He will soon go to sleep so deep that you may do what you wish".

It is difficult to understand how such non-volatile substances were absorbed but that they were used as anaesthetics appears certain.

Mesmerism and hypnotism had been employed by Mesmer and his followers, but the result were very much uncertain.

Syncope was produced by compression of the carotid arteries during very early centuries, but that was also very uncertain.

In 1799 Sir Humphry Davy observed the intoxicating effect of NITROUS OXIDE, which is called as Laughing gas. He thought this gas might benumb a pain and might be used in Surgical operation as an Anaesthetic.

In the year 1815 MICHAEL FARADY observed that ETHER had a similar effect of destroying pain. Within few years "ether frolies" became a quite popular amusement. In 1824 Dr. Henry Hickman of Ludlow Shropshire published his experiment after inhalation of Carbon-di-oxide gas by the animal, a state of unconsciousness and insensibility to pain that was being produced and he throught that this may be taken as a help in Surgery. But it was not taken by the profession and he was called as a "Mad".

After long years in the year 1842 a county practitioner named CRAWFORD LONG (1815-78) participated in an "ETHER FROLIC" and noticed that bruises and minor injuries subtained at the time of Frolics were unaccompanied by pain.

After that he applied Ether to a boy to incise a tumour from the neck in a painless way. All his results and experiments were published in 1849.

In the field of Chemistry GARDNER COLTON, a lecturer in Chemistry made a successful experiment with "LAUGHING GAS" at Hartford.

A local Dentist of Hartford noticed that the victim who inhaled the gas injured his leg in excitement but felt no pain at that time. He persuaded one of his friends Dr. Riggs to use in tooth extraction. Dr. Riggs successfully extracted a Molar tooth. Nitrous Oxide used as an aid for tooth extraction for a short time. But unfortunately it was not popular as WELL failed to show the good result of Nitrous Oxide at all times. Again as Dental anaesthesia in 1890 JOSEPH CLOVER made a reform in the use of Nitrous Oxide. He recommended Nitrous Oxide as preliminary to ETHER ANAESTHESIA.

But the Surgical and dental practitioner preferred Ether as a better one than Nitrous Oxide.

Throughout the world the men of all professions searched out for a good anaesthesia. United States Congress declared an award, but it was not given to anybody as a particular person could not be isolated as the first inventor.

Dec. 21st, 1846 was a remarkable day in the history of Surgery when DR. ROBERT LISTON performed an amputation through the thigh and PETER SMITH administered the anaesthsia. The patient was Fredrick Churchill a Butler of 36 years. The famous witness was JOSEPH LISTER, who was a student at that time.

The benefit of anaesthesia was also taken the Gynae and obst. practitioner. DR. JAMES YOUNG SIMPSON, Professor of Midwifery was also deeply thinking to have some sort of General Anaesthesia for Gynaecological and obsterical purpose. He tried Ether, but the purpose did not serve much.

During this controversal period of Ether regimen in 1831 a Newyork Chemist GUTHRIE discovered a substance called at present as "CHLOROFORM". This was also made independently by SOUBEIRAN and J. VON. LIEBIG.

The substance was named as "CHLOROFORM" and made commercially by M.J. DUMAS of Paris in 1835.

Dr. James Young Simpson took advantage of this substance and used it for Gynaecological purpose, the suggestion came from DAVID WALDIE, a chemist of Liverpool to use it.

The superiority of Chloroform to Eather was noted by Dr. Simpson. On Nov. 10th of 1847 Dr. Simpson communicated his "Account of a new Aneasthetics Agent" to the Edinburg Medical Society. Within five days of the publication of the article Professor Miller of Royal Infirmary removed a part of the Radius suffering from osteomlitis.

For almost half a century chloroform was the choice of anaesthetic for surgical interference in Britain.

DR. JOHN SNOW (1813-58) made extensive researches on the best method of the use of chloroform and wrote a book entitled as - "on Chloroform and other Anaesthetics" in 1858. Dr. Snow was fortunate of administering chloroform to Queen Victoria on two occasions. He was called as the First British Anaesthetist. The ether inhaler he devised is surprisingly modern in design.

He was not only a good anaesthetics but also a pioneer of "PREVENTIVE MEDICINE".

Another London anaesthetic specialist was JOSEPH CLOVER (1825-82) who advised the use of NITROUS OXIDE and ETHER in sequence.

SIR. J. Y. SIMPSON was the first person to use chloroform as anaesthesia. He was the most eminent obstetrician of his days. He was a man of high intellect and distinguished himself as an archaeologist and a pioneer in medicine work by publishing an article on "Leper Hospital in Scotland". He was appointed to the Chair of Midwifery in Edinburg. He discovered a method of "HAEMOSTASIS" by the use of a long needle known as "ACUPRESSURE".

He made notable advances in the technique of ovariotomy and the use of obstetric forecep.

In the British Journal of Anaesthesia 1935, Vol. XII, page 41. A. J. O' Leary raised a question "who was the person who discovered chloroform for anaesthesia"? "Was it Simpson or Waldic"?

Both of them may be given the credit. History will remember both of them.

Simpson's Maternity Hospital now incorporated as part of the Edinburg Royal Infirmary has a bust of the great obstetrician as a memory of his achievement.

The need of ANTENATAL supervision which is now universally recognised was first thought scientifically by a staff of Edinburg obstetrician of Simpson Maternity Hospital, JOHN WILLIAM BALLANTYNE (1861-1923), when in 1889 he presented a thesis for M.D. "MANUAL OF ANTENATAL PATHOLOGY AND HYGIENE" (1902-1904); called the attention of every body.

Every other medical discovery of the 19th century is overshadowed by that of LISTER who by his introduction of the antiseptic method of Surgery, made a complete revolutionary change. By a fortunate coincidence Lister's discovery was made only a few years after the discovery of anaesthesia and the benefit to humanity which followed the introduction of the two methods have been truly uncountable.

Prior to Lister Hospital Gangrene was in an epidemic nature and sepsis was almost an inevitable epidemic of all operations.

Compound fracturers were treated by amputation. The mortality was very high almost 25% to 30%.

The surgeons used to wear an old blood stained coat with a bunch of silk ligatures in the button hole for ready use. There was slow process of healing and odourous pus used to drop down from the wound in a zinc tray.

The patients had to suffer the tortures of operation and later on the agony of pain and danger of Septic wound.

The Supreme Lord move by agony of the surgical patient sent ROBERT LISTON as an angel. ROBERT LISTON (1794-1847) had all the qualifications of a great surgeon.

He was the first in Britain to employ ether anaesthecia when he was

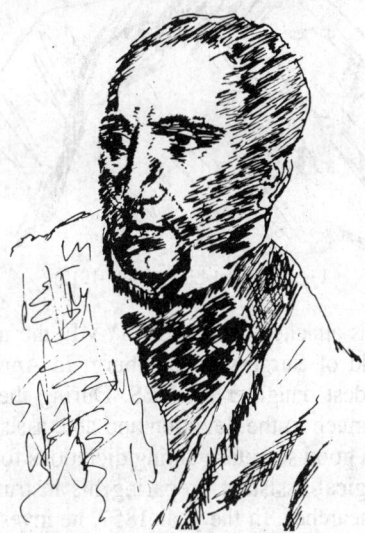

Fig. 50 Robert Liston (1794-1847)

attached at the Uiversity College Hospital of London. He excelled in emergency cases which called for swiftness of decision and originality of Procedure and introduced many novelties, such as popular mode of flap amputation, shoes for club-foot, and his devices for reducing dislocation and crushing and cutting for stone. He was specially successful in plastic operation. In 1837 he described a method of Laryngoscopygin in which he was the early pioneer.

JOSEPH LISTER (1827-1912): ANTISEPTICS

Joseph Lister took his B.A. degree of London before entering university college hospital as a student. He graduated M.B. in year 1852 and later on became a Fellow of the Royal College of Surgeon. He was originally more interested in physiology. His first publication on Physiology was "on Contractile tissues of the Iris", later on published another paper - "Muscular tissue of the skin", the pilomotor fiber which causes "goose skin".

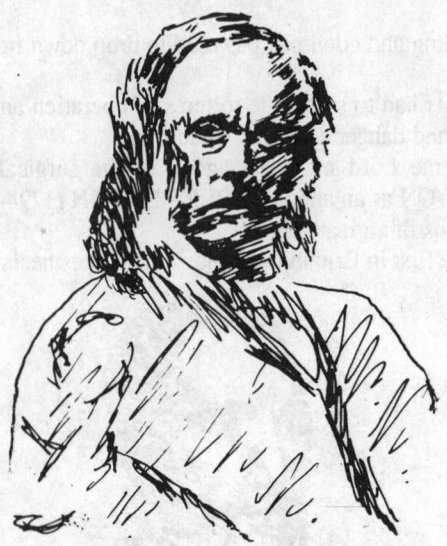

Fig. 51 Lord Lister (1827-1912)

Later on he was attached to JAMES SYME, the most distinguished person in the world of Surgery at Edinburg. In April 23rd, 1856, he married Syme's eldest daughter AGNES. During the next thirty nine years Lister owed much to the devotion and able assistance to his wife, who was not only a good secretary taking dictations for hours and hours but as an able surgical assistant preparing his instrument and a good inspirator to his researches. In the year 1857, he investigated the "early stages of Inflammation in the foot of Frog", and published it in the Royal Society. In the next year he published another paper on the "coagulation of the blood". In 1860 Lister removed to Glasgow the place for his epochmaking discovery.

Lister was appointed as Assistant Surgeon to the Royal Infirmary. His wards in the Glasgow Royal Infirmary was built upon the site of an old burial ground crammed with the coffins of cholera epidemic victim of 1849. Many people attributed the sources of the Hospital gangrene, erysipelas and pyaemia which may be the sources of evils that being carried out from the burial ground.

Lister's researches on inflammation led him to suspect that decomposition and or putrefaction was the cause of suppuration and infection of wounds and the causes are not merely the gases of the air but something carried by the air.

Thomas Anderson, a professor of Chemistry of Glasgow, who drew the attention of Lister of the Pasteur remarks that putrefaction was a

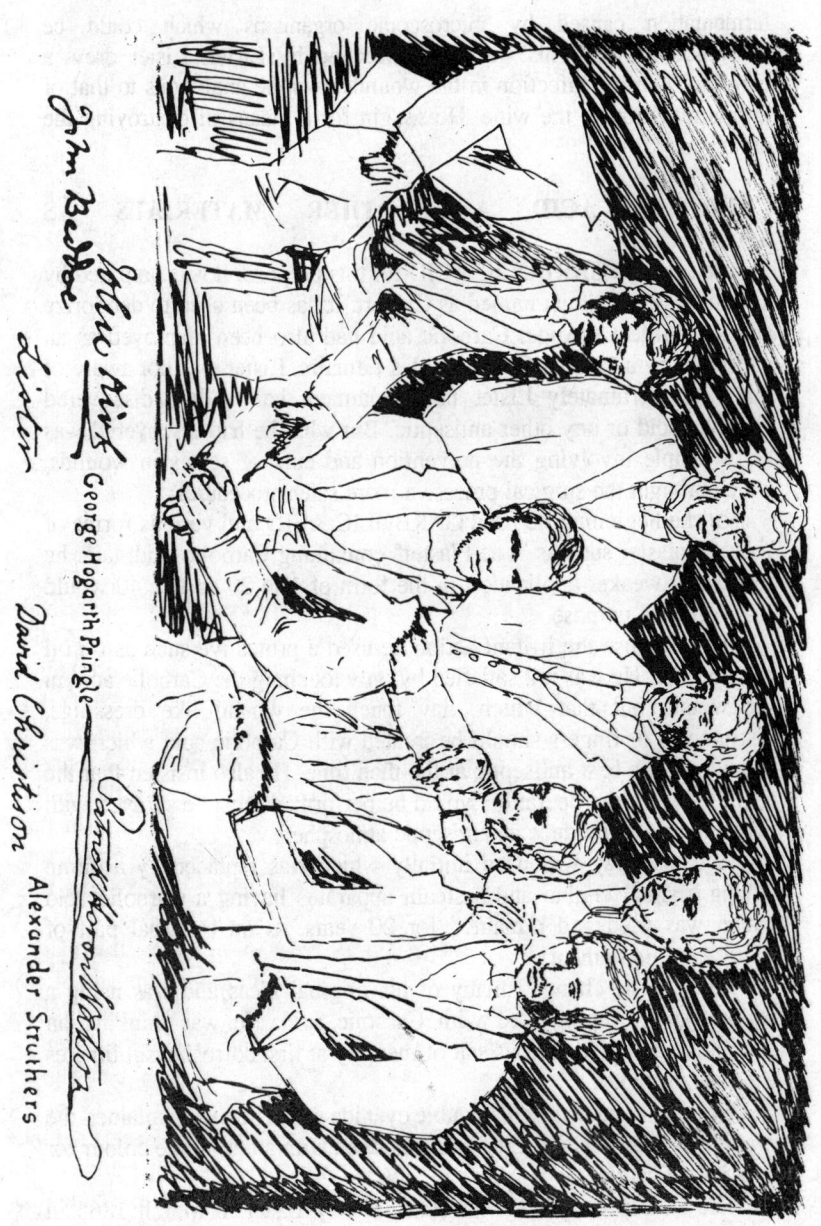

Fig. 52 LISTER AND HIS FELLOW HOUSE-SURGEONS 1854

fermentation caused by microscopic organisms which could be trasmitted by air. This was acknowledged by Lister. Lister drew a corollary that the infection in the wounds must be analogous to that of the putrefaction in the wine. He sought for a means of destroying the organism.

CARBOLIC ACID AND OTHER MATERIALS AS ANTISEPTIC

He selected CARBOLIC ACID for this purpose. It was prepared by a Manchester Chemist named as Calvert. It has been used to deodorize and to disinfect sewage. Carbolic acid had also been employed as an antiseptic by a Persian Chemist Jules Lemaire. Lister was not aware of this fact. Fortunately Lister never claimed that he had discovered Carbolic acid or any other antiseptic. But what he had discovered was the principle involving the prevention and cure of sepsis in wounds, which brought the surgical process a more safer procedures.

At the beginning he used CARBOLIC ACID and various forms of putty or plaster such as "Lac Plaster" containing Carbolic acid, later he found that weaker application in the form of 1 in 20 or 1 in 40 would also serve the purpose.

To minimise the irritant action he used a protective such as tin oil or oiled silk. He was not satisfied by only touching the Carbolic acid in the wound but that which may touch the wound like dressings, instruments or fingers should be treated with Carbolic acid which was considered the best antiseptic at the then time. He also insisted that the room in which the operation would be performed must be sprayed with Carbolic acid to produce an antiseptic atmosphere.

A hand spray was used initially which was replaced by a pump having a small engine and a steam apparatus having a Carbolic acid which was used and remained for 20 years, as an essential part of "Antiseptic Equipment.

Later on he changed many of his original ideas and was using a yellow gauze impregnated with Carbolic acid. He was thinking an alternative and tried various salt of mercury at first corrosive sublimates and then cyanides.

Evantually he favoured "double cyanide gauze" which contained the cyanide of Mercury and Zinc and was dyed with a heliotrope colour for only identification.

The antiseptic system was first used by Lister in March 1865 in treating a compound fracture of the leg. In 1867 he first published his result in The Lancet under "a new method of treating compound Fracture".

While in Edinburg he was holding the Chair of Surgery, after the death of Professor Syme in 1870; during this period he introduced the Carbolic acid spray. He also confirmed the Pasteur's finding that if a boiled urine was kept open in the air but prevented from entering dust by a specially prepared flask with the neck drawn out and twisted; the urine would remain clear. Thus he made a good friendship with Pasture by correspondence only.

He was very minute in detail of the Surgical procedures. He advocated black safety pins for securing bandages and advised these should be inserted parallel to the line of strain.

The SINUS FORCEP and the PROBE-POINTED SCISSORS, which he invented are still used in every hospital.

Two of his favourite sayings were "Success depends upon attention to detail and "There is only rule of practice put yourself in the patients place".

CATGUT

In addition to his immortal works on the prinicple of antiseptic, he introduced CATGUT LIGATURE, because it can be safely put to Carbolic acid. He also introduced RUBBER TUBE drainage; this was introduced by

PIERRE MARIE CHASSAIGNAC, a few years earlier.

His (Lister) first use of the rubber tube drainage was a historical events. It was used when he opened the axillary abscess of QUEEN VICTORIA in 1871 at Balmoral; Sir William Jenner as an assistant helped him to work the bellows of the spray. His antiseptic doctrine was accepted throughout the world.

On February 10th, 1912 at the age of 85 years he died.

With the discovery of the principles of Antiseptic Surgery, all branches of surgical procedures made immense advances.

One of the disciple of Lister was LUCAS CHAMPIONNIERE introduced "Listerism" in France and pioneer in advocating early message and movement in the treatment of Fracture.

There were also leading surgeons in France and pioneer in advocating early message and movement in the treatment of Fracture.

There were also leading surgeons and gynaecologist, anaesthetic in France who introduced many new things in France. Among these were JULES Pean (1830-1898) for performing ovariotomy. Paul Reclus (1874-1914) for local anaesthesia. Marin Theodore Tuffier (1857-1929) for spinal anaesthesia.

Among the Listerian the followers in Germany were Karl Thiersch (1822-95) who devised the method of Skin Grafting.

Actually in the last phase of Lister, 19th century medicine and all other allied branches progressed much. Basic science in branches of Physiology, Biology, heredity and Genetic brought revolutionary thoughts.

ERNST VON BERGMANN (1836-1907) of Riga Russia was equally notable for introducing "STEAM STERILIZATION" in surgery and established the present standardized a septic ritual; with the increase idea of aspectic surgery. He greatly advanced the cranial surgery and was notable for works on fatty embolosism.

The Swiss Surgeon THEODORE KOCHER (1841-1917) revolutionized the surgery of Thyroid gland. The Italian Surgeon EDWARDO BASSI (1844-1924) evolved a modernised technique of the operation of Inguinal herina.

In British Isles SIR JONATHAN HUTCHISON (1828-1913) a contemporaries of Lister was a man of encyclopaedic knowledge. He made valuable contribution on Syphilis and Leprosy.

The Gynaeocological Surgery also advanced very fast. The name of Sir Spencer Wells and Robert Lauson Tait were well remembered by us. In America HOWARD KELLY of Baltimore (1858-1943) was a leading Gynaecological Surgeon. He introduced the USE OF RADIUM.

Along with the advancement of Surgical procedures; Surgical pathology gradually came up. Many eminent physcians contributed their best in this field of Pathology.

PAGET SURGICAL PATHOLOGY

SIR JAMES PAGET (1814-99) of England was a great SURGICAL PATHOLOGIST like BRODIE.

HUTCHINSON

SIR JONATHAN HUTCHINSON (1828-1913) of Youkrshire, a great surgical Pathologist is specially remembered for his description of the NOTCHED, PEGSHAPED INCISOR TEETH (HUTCHINSON'S TEETH) IN CONGENITAL SYPHILIS (1861); and of Varicella Gangrenosa (1882).

His name is further associated with the "HUTCHINSON'S FACIES" in opthalmoplegia, "HUTCHINSON'S MASK" in Tabes, the unequal pupils in meningeal haemorrhage and "HUTCHISON'S TRIAD" the enterstial Keratitis, notched teeth, labyrinthine disease in syphilis.

In this period in America there were eminent surgeon like HENRY JACOB BIGELOW (1816-90) as an Orthopaedic surgeon who described the mechanism of iliofemoral or Y ligament and its importance in reducing dislocation of Hip joint by flexion method. SAMUEL DAVID GROSS (1805-84) and WILLIAM KEEN successfully tapped the ventricles of the brain JHON THOMPSON HODGEN (1826-62) who devised the wire suspension splints for fracture of the femur and foream, and CHARLES Mc BURNEY (1845-1913). Who devised the so-called "GRIDIRON INCISION" and discovered the "Mc. BURNEY'S point's as a sign of operative intervention in appendicitis.

*and operated in a case of meningioma, who lived thirty years after operation.

GYNAECOLOGY: The Gynaecology of the post listerian period had a brilliant development of the operative principles, which have been established by Mc. Dowell, SIMS, EMMETT AND BATTEY in America, KOEBERLE in France GUSTAV SIMON in Germany and SIR THOMAS SPENCER WELLS (1818-97) in England and ROBERT LAWSON TAIT (1845-99) of Edinburg. All were of huge reputations for female patients seeking operative relief.

Along with the others were HOWARD ATWOOD KELLY of Philadelphia for introducing Nephro-ureterectomy, nephro-ureterocystectomy, vertical bisection of uterus in Hysterectomy, operating on the Kidney by the superior lumbar Triangle, treatment of malignant Tumors by Radium. The ETIENNE TARNIER of Paris was also famous as inventor of AXIS-TRACTION FORCEP.

OBSTETRIC FORCEP

There are a few names of modern times which must be remembered. They were SIMPSON; CREDE, BRAXTON HICKS, Sir James Yuong SIMPSON; CREDE, BRAXTON HICKS, long obstetric forcep, uterine sound, the sponge test and "SIMPSON PAIN" in uteri cancer. Carl Siegmund Franz CREDE (1819-92) of Berlin introduced two things of capital importance. His methods of removing PLACENTA by EXTERNA MANUAL EXPRESSION and preventing GONORRHEAL INFANTILE CONJUNCTIVITIS by instillation of Silver Nitrate Solution into the eyes of newborn.

John Braxton HICKS (1825-67) of London made an epoch in the history of obstetric procedure by introducing of PODALIC version by combined external and internal manipulation.

OPTHALMOLOGY

HERMANN VON HELMHOLTZ (1821-94)—A professor of Physiology and Pathology at Knoigsberg and ultimately a Professor of Physics at Berlin, was a man of outstanding personality and versatile genius.

His invention of OPTHALMOSCOPE made opthalmology an exact Science (1851). It was follwed by PHAKOSCOPE and OPTHALMOMETER (1852) with the latter he was able to determine the optical constant and explain the mechanism of accommodation particularly the part played by the lens.

The physical theory of vision which might be said as the ground work of opthamology was due to the works of great astronomers and physicists.

"The Ad vitellionem Paralipomena" of the astronomer KEPLER (1604) contained a description on vision and the human eye in which he showed for the first time how retina is essential to sight and the part the lens played in refraction and the convergence of luminous rays before reaching the retina in the cause of MYOPIA.

EDME MARIOTTE (Died 1684) proved that a luminous eye is due to reflection of light and discovered the blind spot in the retina (1668).

In 1587 ARANZI demonstrated the reversal of the image projected on the retina in cattle and had shown the lateral entry of the optic nerve.

To trace out the detail history of opthalmology one has to go back to 16th century and should keep in mind GEORGE BARTISCH an unlettered barber surgeon, who showed certain procedures in cataract operation.

In the 17th century the physical theory of vision which might be called the ground work of OPTHALMALOGY the credit goes to the great number of astronomers and physicists. "The ADVITELIONEM, PARALIPOMENA" a treatise on vision was written by the astronomer KEPLER (Frank Fort 1604). It contained writings on vision and of human eye in which he has shown for the first time part played by lens for refraction and that the convergence of Luminous rays of light before reaching the retina is the cause of "Myopia".

In "DIOPTRICA" treatise written by RENE DESCARTES, the eye, was compared with a camera and the accommodation of the eye is mainly controlled by the changes on the lens.

EDME MARIOTTE discovered the blind spot in the retina. The Jesuit astronomer CHRISTOPH SCHEINER was a remarkable pioneer in the physiologic optic.

In 1619 SCHEINER in his treatise "OCULUS" gave an ingenious demonstration of how images ball on the human retina noticed the changes in curvature of the lens during accommodation and illustrated accommodation and refraction by the pin hole test, which bears in his name.

In the 18th century, remarkable contribution and lectures were made by HERMANN BOER HAAVE (1668-1732) in the subject of opthalmalogy.

The surgery of the eye owes one of its telling advancements to JACQUES DAVIEL (1696-1762). He was the originator of the Modern treatment of cataract by extraction of the lens.

The important facts of the clouding and hardening of lens was brought out by BRISSEAU (1706) and MALTRE-JAN (1707).

In 1672 "MAITRE-JAN proved by post mortem that the particular type of opacity in the lens was cataract, not the skin or any pellicle in the lens was cataract, not a nost of skin or any pellicle inside the capsul. JACQUES DAVIEL within few years of introducing his modern treatment of cataract by extraction of the lens, he (DAVIEL) had a record of 434 extractions with only 50 failures, from that time his method became a permanent procedure in opthalmic surgery, only additional modification of ioidectomy was made VON GRAFFE.

One of the outstanding figures in the history of opthalmalogy was

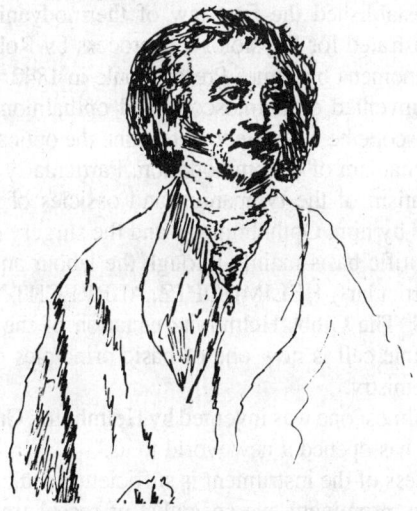

Fig. 54 Thomas Young (1773-1829)

THOMAS YOUNG (1773-1829) of Milverton, England. He qualified his M.B. and M.D. at Cambridge in the year 1803 and 1808.

In the year 1792 he said the visual accommodation of the eye at different distances is due to change of curvature in the crystalline lens. In 1801 he gave in detail the description of astigmatism with measurements and optical constant. He also stated the present YOUNG HELMHOLTZ theory that colour vision is due to retinal structures corresponding with red green, violet and the colour blindness is due to deficient response of these to normal stimuli in the retina.

In 1808 Young clearly stated the laws governing the flow of blood in the Heart and arteries.

As a man of science particularly in physics Thomas Young was most famous as the author of Wave theory of light. In 1809 he showed its application to crystalline refraction and dispersion phenomena. which led to the Fresnel theory of double refraction (1821) and the Helmholtz theory of dispersion for absorbent media.

In the second half of 19th century there were masters in Physiology like HERMANN VON HELMHOLTZ. CLANDE BERNARD and CARL LUDWIG.

VON HELMHOLTZ (1820-1894) of Potsdam was a product of German. English and French culture. In 1842, he made a disertation lecture dealing with the origin of never fifers from cells in the ganglia of leaches and crabs, which he observed with a rudimentary compound microscope. Helmholtz gave universal application of conservation of energy which established the first law of thermodyanics; which was actually demomstrated for Physiological process by Robert Mayer and for physical Phenomena by James Prescot Joule in 1842.

Helmholtz invented opthalmoscope and opthalmometer. With the latter and phakoscope he was able to determine the optical constants and explain the mechanism of accommodation. Particularly part played by the lens Mechanism of the tympanum and ossicles of the middle ear was also studied by him. Opthalmology and the surgery of the eye were put upon a scientific basis mainly through the labour and contributions of three men particularly HELIMHOPTZ. ALBRECHT VON GRAEFE and DONDERS. The Gibbs-Helmholtz equation of the electro-motive force of a galvanic cell is now one of basic principles of physical and phyiological chemistry.

When opthalmoscope was invented by Helmholtz; Graefe exclaimed that "Helmholtz has opened a new world to us."

The usefulness of the instrument is sufficiently indicated by the fact that nearly every prominent eye specialist of recent times has tried to add some improvement to it. Not only did it indicate the disorders of the unveal tract, but even such obscure diseases as those of brain, the kindeys, and the pituitary body.

Before the time of Von graefe, the infectious forms of granular conjunctivitis had been described by Boron Larrey (1802), John Vetch (1807) and Jacob Christian Bendz (1855), WILLIAM HYDE WOLLASTON had invented periscopic spectacles (1803) and the camera lucida (1807); Benjamin Gibson had demonstrated that ophthalmia neonatorum is due to the vaginal secretions (1807) and the possibility of couching cataract in the new-born (1811); hyoscyamin and atropin had been used in examination by Franz Reisinger (1825); Sir George Airy had described astignmatism (named by who well; test readings of print of a distance had been employed by J. Ayscough (1752), J.G.A Cchevallier (1805), G. Tauber (1816), F. Holke (1830), F. Cunier (1841), and K. Himly (1843); Eduard types were introduced by Heinrich Kuchler (Schrif tnummer probe, 1843); Eduard Jaeger Von Jaxthal (1854), C. Stellwag von Carion (1855), Grafe and Donders (1860), Hermann Snellen (1862), Ezra Dyer (1862), Giraud Teulon (1862), and J. Green (1866-1868). Kussmaul had described the colour phenomena in the fundus (1854); J. Mery (1704), Purkinje (1823), William Cumming (1846), and Ernst Brucke (1847), had considered the significance of luminosity of the eye in vertebrates and man; Philip Franz von Walther had described corneal opacity (1845); and Ernst Bricke (1847), and Sichel had published his spectales (1802), the mechanism of vision had been studied by Thomas (1845) and a good treatises on eye disease had been written by Antonic Scarpa (1801), James Wardrop (1808), George Joseph Beer (1813-17), Benjamin Travers (1820), John Vetch (1920), George Firck (Baltimore (1824), William Mackenzie (1830), Sir William Lawrence (1833), Squier Littell (Philadelphia, 1836 C-J-F-Carrdu villards (1838) Friedrich August von Ammon (1838-1) the Canadian Henry Howard (1850), Karl Himly (1843), Louis- Auguste, Desmarres (1847), Carl Stellwag von Carion (1853-1858) and Carl Ferdinand Von Arlt (1851-41). The surgery of the eye had been advanced by George James Guthrie (1823), J.F. Dieffenbach (Strabismus 1842), Thomas Wharton Jones (1847), L-A Desmarres (1850) and particularly by Sir William Bowman (artifical pupil 1852); lacrimal obstruction 1857). In 1820 Captain Charles Barbier laid before the Academie des science a monograph on teachng the blind to and write by a system of combinations of six elevated points instead of embossed lines. The Barbier six point system was introduced in paris by Louie Braille, a blind teacher of the in 1820 and in 1836 Braille introduced his system of musical notation for the blind. He acknowledged his indebtedness to Captain CHARLES Barbier in the preface to his book (1837). In 1845-1847 William Moon, of Brighton, England introduced the Roman line types which are still used. but by 1879, the Barbier Braille types had become a world alphabet for the blind.

A.V. GRAEFE

Albrecht von Graefe (1828-70) of Berlin, the creator of the modern surgery of the eye and indeed the greatest of all eye surgeons, was the son of Carl Ferdinand von Graefe. After graduating in Berlin in 1847, he was urged to specialize in ophthalmology by Arlt in prague, and having followed the clinics of Sichel and Desmarres in Paris, the Jaegers in Vienna, Bowman and Crishett in London. He soon obtained phenomenal success in the native city. He became the professor at the university in 1857. In 1854, he founded the Archiv fur Ophthalmologie, has remained the leading organ of specialty to date. The first volume of his book alone contains his papers on the disorders of the oblique eye muscles. The nature of glaucoma, keratoconus, mydriasis, diphtheritic conjunctivitis, and on double vision after strabismus operations.

Von Graefe introduced the operation of iridectomy in the treatment of iritis, iridochoriditis and glaucoma (1855-62) made the operation for strabismus viable (1871) and improved the treatment of cataract by the modified linear extraction (1845-68) which reduced the loss of the eye from 10 to 2.3 per cent. He applied the ophthalmoscope to the study of the amblyopias in functional disorders with extraordinary success, made a brilliant diagnosis of embolism of the retinal artery as the cause of a sudden blindness (1850) and proceeded to point out that most cases of blindness and impaired vision connected with cerebral disorders are traceable to optic neurits rather than to paralysis of the optic nerve (1860) the view manitained before his time. Graefe was also the founder of modern knowledge of sympathetic opthalmia and the semeiology of ocular paralysis and described conical cornea, or "Keratoconus" (1854) and first noted the stationary condition of the upper eyelid when the eyeball is rolled up or down, in exophthalmic goiter (Graefe's sign 1864). His pupils included nearly all the greatest ophthalmologists of the 19th century.

Frams Cornelius Donders (1818-89) of Tilburg, Holland, was educated as an army surgeon, but became a professor in the Utrecht Faculty in 1848, and after 1862, devoted himself exclusively to ophthalmology.

To this field belong his studies of the muscae volitantes (1847) the use of prismatic glasses in strabisnus (1848) the relation between convergence of visual axes and accommodation (1848), hypermetropia (1858-60), ametropia and its sequels (1860), astigmatism (1862-3), anomalies of refraction as a cause of strabismus (1863) and above all his great work on the Anomalies of Refraction and Accommodation, which was published not in Dutch, but in English, by the New Sydenham society (1864). As a contribution to physiological optics, this book rank with the labour of Helmholtz. It contains Donders explanation of astigmatism, his definitions of aphakia and hypermetropi, his sharp distinctions between myopia and hypermetropia (as errors of refraction) and presbyopia (as senile change with diminished accommodation). His views of myopia as the result of excessive convergence and the cause of genuine divergent strabismus, of hypermetropia as the cause of convergent strabismus, of the ciliary muscle as the only muscle use in accommodation and its action in bulging the anterior surface of the lens, and of asthenopia (eye-strain) as the result of anomalies of refraction, muscular insufficiency or astigmatism.

Donders work has been the main source of knowledge on the improvement of disorders of vision by spectacles upto the time of Gullstrand. It is said that while impatiently writing for one of Helmholtz's ophtalmoscopes, he contrived one for himself in which the silvered mirror with central perforation, now in use was substituted for the superimposed glass plates of the Berlin Master's instrument. Landesh Gasthuis voor Oogleiden). But his labors were not entirely confined to the eye. His most important contribution to physiology was the first measurement of the reaction time of a psychical process. (1868). In 1845 he wrote on the physiology of speech (1864-70). Donders was highly accomplished in speaking English, French and German like a native, yet modest to the point of diffidence. His earlier military avocations gave him a polished tenure which with his natural personal charm made him known all over Europe as one of the most attractive specialists of his time.

ALFRED KARL GRAEFI

Prominent among von Craefe's pupils were his nephew, Alfred Karl Graefe (1830-99) who made a clinical analyais of disordered movements of the eye (1858), invented a special localization ophthalmoscope for extractiing deep-lying cysticerci. He wrote a monograph on the treatment of infantile conjunctivitis by caustics and antiseptics (1881) and with Saemisch edited the well-known Graefe Saemisch "Hand buch der Ophthalmologic" (1874-80). JULIUS JACOBSON (1828-89) of Konigberg who made a great improvement in the operative treatment of cataract by his peripheral incision under chloroform anesthesia (1853) reducing the loss of the eye from 10 to 2 percent and further improving the operation by extraction within the capsule (1888) original the operative treatment of tiachoma and trichiasis (1887). He wrote a fine memoir on the work of his friend von Craefe (1885) and enjoyed the largest consulting practice on eastern Europe, patients streaming in even from Russia; the brother Alexander (1828-79) and Hermaon Pagenstecher (1844-1918) the former of whom made his mark in the history of cataract by the extraction of the lens in the closed capsule through a scleral incision (1866). EDWIN THEODER SAEMISCH

(1833-1909) of Luckau, who first described serpiginous ulcer of the cornea and its treatment (1870) and vernal conjunctivitis (1876) and edited a handbook with the younger Graefe; THEODOR LEBER (1840-1917) who studied the diabetic disorders of the eye (1875) and the disorders of circulation and nutrition of the eye (1876). Richard Liebreich (1830-1917) of Konigsberz who introduced lateral illumination in microscopic investigation of the living eye (1855) and published by Jaeger von Jaxtthal (1869) and Hermann JAKOB KNAPP who became one of the leading opthalmologist of New York City, founded the Archives of Ophthalmology and otology (New York 1869) and wrote valuable memoirs on curvature of the cornea (1859) and intra ocular turmors (1860) and other subjects.

On the detective side the most eminent ophthalmologist is ERUST FUCHS (1851-?) of Vienna a pupil of Bruke and Billroth Arlt's assistant (1870-80) professor of ophthalmology at Liege (1880-85) and Vienna (1885). His is the author of important monographs on sarcoma of the uveal tract (1882), blindness (1885), and the histopathology of sympathetic ophthalmia (1905), of improvements of Jaegor's test-types (Leseproben fur die Nahe 1895) and of the standing German treatise on eye diseases (1889) which was passed through 12 editions and many translations, including the Japanese.

Of work relating to the normal eye, we may mention Henry Gray's memoir on the optic nerves (1849), Max Schultze's memoir on the anatomy and physiology of the retina (1866), the theories of vision of Helmholtz (1867), Ewald Hering (1872) and Christine Ladd Franklin (1882), willy Kuhne's investigations of visual purple (1877) and the memoirs of Ramony Cajal on the vertebrate retina (1895) and of Johannes von kries (1853) on the function of the retinal rods (1895). The examination of the eye was further improved by such inventions as the astigmometer (1967) of Emile Javal (1839-1907) of Paris; by the Javel Schiotz ophthalmometer (1881) by the method of retinosecopy introduced by Ferdinand Cuignet (1873) and by the Kerato-scope invented by A. Placido (1882). Colour blindness was investigated by the Swedish physiologist Alarik Frithi of Holmgren (1831-97) who introduced the wool skein test (1874) and gave special consideration to colour blindness under railway and maritime conditions (1878). The relation of eye-strain (asthenopia) and astigmatism to headaches and other neurotic symptoms was first noted by S. Weir Mitchell, morbid psychology (1888) by George Milbry Gould (1847-1922) who showed that a very minute error of refraction, discoverable only after paralysis of accommodation by cyeloplegics, may suffice to lower resistance to diseases by profound nervous irritation and mental misery strainmay be due to congenital malformation of the sclera (Arthur Keith). The work of Alexender Duane (1858-1926) on refraction (1916) has taught much. The relation of eye diseases to general and organic diseases of the body was especially treated by Richard Forster (1877) and in 1898 by Hermann Schmidt-Rimpler (1838-1915) who was also with Hermann Cohn (1838-1906) a pioneer in the examination of the eyes of School childern. The semeiology of the eye in nervous diseases was treated inextenso by Hermann Wilbrandt and Alfred Sanger (1900-1913). The bacteriology of the eye was especially advanced by Robert Koch who discovered the bacilli of two different forms of Egyptian conjunctivitis (1883) by John E. Weeks who found the same organism as the cause of Pink-eye (1886); by Henri Parinaud (1844-1905) of Paris who described an infectious tubercular conjunctivitis transmissible from animals to man (1880) and a lacrimal pneumococcic conjunctivitis in newborn infant (1874) both associated with his name; and by Victor Morax and Theodor Axenfeld who simulataneously described the diplobacillary from of chornic conjunctivitis (1896-97). In 1894 Axenfeld described the pyemicor metastatic opthalmia first noted by J. H. Meckel in 1854. Apart from the Graefe Saemisch Handbook, the best modern works on ophthalmology are the monumental treatises of Ernst Funchs (1880-1920) with 12th edition and Louis de Wecker (1832-1906) and Edmond Landolt (1846-1926) whose name is especially associated with an operation of congenital and paralytic ptosis (1886). Besides the Americans already referred to we may mention Henry Willard Williams (1821-1895) who introduced the treatment of iritis without mercury (1856) and a method of suturing the flap after cataract extraction (1866); Cornelius Rea Agnew (1830-88) who described a method of operating for divergent squint (1866); Henry Drury Noyes (1832-1900) was the author of the Muscles of the Eye (1907). Casey A. Wood (1856-?) editor of the American Encylopedia of Ophthalmology (1913-21) notable for work on alcoholic amblyopia (1904) and a monograph on the fundus oculi in birds (1917); Edward Jackson (1856-?) editor of the American Journal of Ophthalmology (1898) author of a valuable work on skiascopy (1892) who has done much valuable work on the toxic amblyopias (1896) and the work of E. Dyer on asthenopia (1865), George T. Stevens on Classification of the heterophorias (1886), G. C. Savage on functions of the oblique muscles (1893) and William H. Wilmer on eye conditions in aviators (1918), many instruments and test types have been invented notably the electric light ophthalmoscope of W. S. Demnett. F. Buler's shield for ophthalmia neonatorum (1874) and the tangent-plane of Alexander Duane.

During end of 19th century, the leading English neurologists of the period who made remarkable contribution in the field of opthalmology were JOHN HUGHLINGS JACKSON (1834-1911) and WILLIAM RICHARD GWOERS (1845-1915), Jackson stressed much to establish the use of the opthalmoscope in the diagnosis of brain diseases. Similarly Gower also did much to connect the diseases of the central nervous system and the eye. His treatise on medical opthalmology was written in the year 1897 and was of much help to the professional people.

The NOBEL PRIZE of 1911 in medicine was awarded to ALLVAR GULISTRAN of Landsknona Sweden professor of Opthalmology for his valuable contribution. In the University of Upsala (1804), Gullstrand made his mathematical investigations of dioptrics or the science of the refraction of light through the transparent media of the living eye. As Willard Gibbs founded the Chemical theory of heterogenous substances, so Gullstrand has founded the dioptrics of heterogeneous media.

Formerly, the image in the eye was regarded as a schematic, "co-linear", or point-for-point arrangement, like that studied on the lenses of optical instruments. The course of the rays in astigmatism. For instance, was represented by the dia-grammatic Sturm's conoid. Gullstrand took up the study of the ocular image from the viewpoint of reality, clearly differentiating its actual formation from its optical projection. He showed that the assemblage of rays in sturm's conoid had not the slightest resemblance to the actual condition in astigmatism. By applying the methods of mathematical physics, especially those of Sir William Rowan Hamilton, (1828) he treated the problem as one concerning a set of widely diffused bundles of rays, refracted through a system of continually curving planes, and showed that, during accommodation the index of refraction of the lens is augmented by an actual change in its structure.

His principal works on this theme are his study of astigmatism (1891), his General Theory of Monochromatic Aberrations (1900) and his essays on dioptrics of the crystalline lens (1906) and the real optic image (1906) are very important in the field of opthalmology. In 1889 he introduced a practical method of estimating corneal astingmatism by a single observation, an advantage possessed by a single instrument, the sutcliffe opthalmometer. In 1802 he introduced a photographic method of locating a paralyzed ocular muscle. He also introduced a micrometric method of estimating the photo-graphed corneal reflex, as giving the most exact knowledge of the form of the normal and diseased cornea. His work in the field is not unlike Burdon-sanderson's photographic that the yellow colour of the macula in the retina is a cadaveric phenomenon, not existing in life; and he discovered the intracapsular mechanism of accommodation. He also devised the reflexless stationary opthalmoscope (1912), which excludes all light not belonging to the opthalmoscopic image and is thus free from all relfections from the mirror or the itself, giving a better image, better streoscopic effect and a wider field aspherical lenses for those operated on for contract, which give cleaner cut and more luminous images, with wider range of vision, than spherical lenses with the same focal distance, and laterly the slit-lamp (1902) which permits of microscopic study of the living eye.

Two prominent innovations in eye surgery of recent times times have been made by officers of the Indian Medical Service. The operation of extraction of cataract within the capsule was introduced by COLONEL HENRY SMITH in 1900, and his success with it has been remarkable. As a benefector of humankind, he is known allover northern India, where the reflection of the pitiles sunlight from the dusty plains tells with terrific force upon the eye of the natives.

His clinics at Jullundur and Amritsar, in the Punjab, are frequented not only by stream of blind people coming by every mode of travel but by opthalmic surgeons, even from the western United States who travel across the world to learn his methods. He teaches by making the pupil perform the operation before him. He averages about 3000 extractions a year, and by 1910, he had 24,000 to his credit, of which 20,000 were done by the intracapsular method. Another new operation, that of sclerocorneal trephining for glaucoma, was introduced by MAJOR ROBERT HENRY ELLIOT, I.M.S. in August, 1909. The operation of von Graefe had held the field for half a century; Lagrange and Herbert had emphasized the value of sclerectomy, and even corneal trephining had been essayed by Argyll Robertson, Blanco, Frohlich, and Freeland Fergus, but Elliot had made the operation his own by many improvements and has made it viable. Latterly, diathermy and protein-therapy have proved effective weapons in the management of diseases of the eye.

BACTERIOLOGY

It is very difficult to say, when to start and where to start the history and importance of bacteriology in matters medical.

Since the birth of a life, man wanted to negate death. To find out the real cause of death, a condition known as "disease process" was noted.

Intially disease was considered as a displeasure of God or an influence of an evil spirit or morbid materials. So it was thought that death is a punishment for disobedience.

In certain sector of the globe there was a belief that man was at one time capable of renewing his youth by casting the skin but the process should be taken in secret. Once an old man indiscretly allowed his grand daugther to witness the operation and thus the displeasure of God aroused and the benefit was withdrawn. Similarly "eating of the forbidden fruit brought death into World" were also considered.

From the time of Hippocrates—Aristotle-Galen, Avicenna, men tried to draw a harmonious relation between cause and effect, and drew up certain measures to fight out the sufferings. With the evolution of sciences in all its branches and with improved instrumental aid from the days of Antaoj van Leuwenhoek the attempts were partially successful. Without any assumption these instrumental aids have proved the existence of very minute animated beings as a probable cause of diseases.

Advancement of Pathology and Bacteriology almost went side by side. In the 19th century the motto in Pathology was "OMINS CELLULA E CELLUA" and this was the foundation of work of CEllular pathology made by VIRCHOW (RUDOLE VIRCHOW-1821-1902). So the primitive men did not attempt to find out the cause the disease process. No attempt was to solve the riddle of the disease made. The discovery of bacteria caused a many change in the knowledge of diseased's processes (pathology), especially in the later part of the 19th century.

The greatest exponents of Pathology, specially in the 19th century was CARL ROKITANSKY (1804-78) a czech who was a professor of Pathology at vienna and RUDOLF VIRCHOW (1821-1902).

Contemporary was a Frenchman—LOUIS PASTEUR and the great German ROBERT KOCH.

These two were the founders of bacteriology. Louis Pasteur was not only the founder of bacteriology but was the pioneer of preventive medicine also. Reobert Koch developed the theory of specific infections diseases and went a further step.

Before the time of Pasture, small animated life was also found out by Leuwenhoek who had seen the Protozoa (1675) and bacteria (1687) under the microscope. AGOSTINO Bass found out the presence of microorganism in a diseased silk worm fortunately, and Sarcinae was found out in the stomach by JOHN GOODSIR.

In 1773 and 1786 OTTO FRIEDRIK MULLER was first to classify bacteria and protozoa. In 1778 C.F. VON GLEICHEN attempted to stain the bacteria and protozoa with indigo and carninu, this methods were more detailed out by C.G. EHRENBERG, where he had included vibrio, spirillum and spirochoeta in the classification;

cultivation of these small animated life was first made on POTATO as solid media by FRESENIUS in 1863.

In 1869 and 1875 HOFFMANN and SCHROTER first indentified the bacteria by their cultural characteristic which made FERDINAND JULLIUS CHON to have a morphological classification of bacteria.

Though it was not under the domain of medicine yet these invention made by the Bio scientist had helped the bacteriologist, to utilise these knowledges in the field of medicine.

He identified the spores in bacillus subtiles. Before Koch there were certain remarkable works done by KRICHER (1658), PLENCIZ (1762), HENLE (1840). They announced the theory of "CONTAGIUM ANIMATUM".

In 1846 HERMANN KLENCKE had demonstrated that Tuberculosis may be transmitted by cow's milk. It is also interesting to know that JEAN-ANTOINE-VILLEMIN had demonstrated that "tubucular virus" is specific and inoculable which was confirmed by Edwin Kleb (1873), L.A. Thaon and J.J. Grancher and Julius Cohnheim.

Contemporary with Virchow there was a frenchman, who though not a medical graduate, but was one of the outstanding figure in the medical history-LOUIS PASTEUR (1822-1895). He had a great aptitude in drawing portraits but his inquisite mind made him to investigate diseases of wine, insects, domestic animals and ultimately of mankind.

Pasteur was a professor of Chemistry at Strassburg, at Lille and at Paris. The last six years of his life was spent in an Institute, which was named after him in 1888. His first research was an "Crystallography" and he noted how fermentation occurred which led him to study of the causes of putrefaction and fermentation.

He was showed that fermentation was not merely a chemical reaction but was due to some Microorganism.

When he was at Lille a wine district, he discovered that it was the action of organism that caused the wine and milk to become sour and that could be prevented by heat or known as "Pasteurization". These organism were not presented in the substance but had the proof of existence in the atmospheric germs.

This theory helped Lister to use in surgery with amazing results. When Silkworm disease made an havoc in France, Pasture discovered that the Silk worm of two distinct type of diseases and advocated certain measures to prevent it.

To prevent Anthrax or splenic fever, following the line laid down by Jenner, Pasture prepared a weak form of virus, and old culture of low virulence which when injeced into an animal, caused a mild attack and conferred immunity. A similar means was devised for the prevention of chickenpox, cholera.

His famous discovery was made on July 6, 1885 when he treated a boy named JOSEPH MEISTER, who had been bitten by a mad dog. A few months later Pasture had a second successful case when he inoculated a shepherd lad from the Jura named Jupille who had been bitten severly by a rabid dog.

After many years of research Pasture came to the conclusion that the virus which causes the Rabies in animals and Hydrophobia in man had its seat in the nerve centres. From the spinal marrow he produced an atternuated virus for inoculation and the success of his bold experiment which led to the establishment of Pasture institutes in many parts of the world and to reduce the morality to less than a percent.

Pasture had many students, among them ELIE METCHNIKOFF

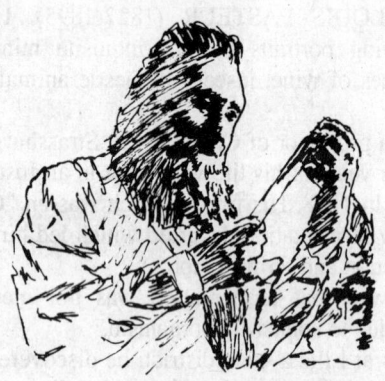

Fig. 56 Elie Metchnikoff (1845-1916)

(1845-1916) the Russian Scientist to whom the nobel prize was awarded in 1908 while he was working at the Marine laboratory of Messina.

He investigated on the digestive process in the larva starfish and planarian worms, which led him to establish the theory of Phagocytosis, the destruction of bacteria, by white blood corpuscle. He received nobel prize in 1908.

The major works of Pasture have been inscribed over his tomb, the molecular dyssymmetry (1848) fermentations (1857), Spontaneons generation (1862), diseases of the wine (1863), diseases of silkworms (1865), microorganism in beer (1871), virulent diseases (anthrax. Chicken pox, Cholera-1877), preventive vaccinations (1880), molecular dyssymmetry (1848) fermentations (1857), Spontaneons generation (1862), diseases of the wine (1863), diseases of silkworms (1865), microorganism in beer (1871), virulent diseases (anthrax. Chicken pox, Cholera-1877), preventive vaccinations (1880), particularly hydrophobia (1885).

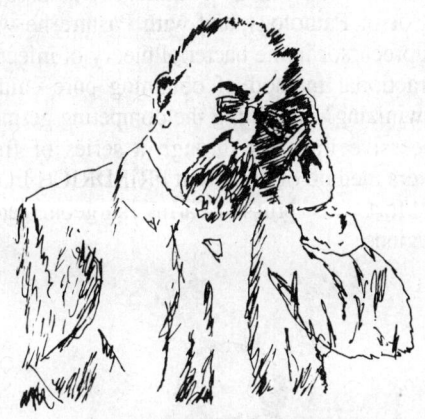

Fig. 57 Robert Koch (1843-1910).

Next to mention is the ROBERT KOCH (1843-1910) the great German pioneer who shared with Pasture as the title of the founder of Bacteriology.

He showed that Anthrax, which was so prevalent in animals and man at that time, was due to large bacillus which has been discovered by POLLENDER in 1849 and was not the result of such vague causes as "Miasmata" or "Contagia". He published his result in 1876 the real cause of Anthra.

In Koch's opinion, the specificity of an organism could only be accepted when certain facts known as "KOCH'S PASTULE" were established in 1881. The germ must be invariably present and must be capable of cultivation outside the body and if injected into the healthy animal reproduces the disease.

Koch discovered the "VIRUS of CHOLERA" in 1884 and showed how it was transmitted by drinking water.

In 1882 he announced the discovery "TUBERCLE BACILLUS" and in 1890 he suggested a new remedy consisting of glycerine extract of tubercle bacillus which he called "TUBERCULIN".

He received many honours including nobel prize in 1905.

Pasteur was succeeded by his assistant "EMILE ROUX" 1853 to 1933 a great French bacteriologist. He perfected the preparation of "ANTI DIPHTHERITIC SERUM" and showed that monkeys could be "INOCULATED with SYPHILIS".

Another well known bacteriologist of Paris, who first applied in 1886 the "SERO-DIAGNOSTIC TEST FOR TYPHOID FEVER" which bears his name -GEORGES WIDAL (1862-1929).

EDWIN KLEBS (1834-1913) of Konigsberg, East Prussia was an eminent professor of Pathology and with Pasture he was perhaps the most important precursor in the bacterial theory of infection in 1874 He invented the fractional method of obtaining pure culture of bacteria known as "Darwinizing" i.e. killing the competing germs in the impure culture by successive transfers through a series of fresh media and followed by listers method of dilutation FRIEDRICH LOFFLER (1852-1915) of Frankfort was prussian army surgeon, later on became Professor of Hygiene.

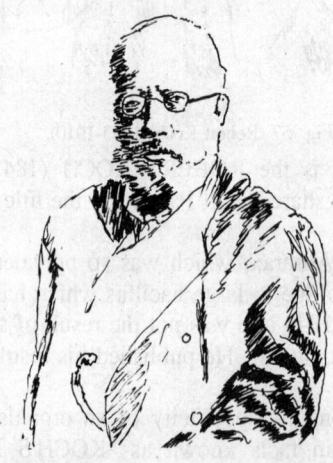

Edwin Klebs (1834–1913).

He invented the swine erysipelas (1882-83) and glanders (1882) and established the causal relation of Diptheria bacillus differentiating it from psuedo-Diptheritia organism and eradicated the field mouse plague in Thessaly by means of Bacillus typhi murium and his investigation of the foot and mouth disease; he was able to prove experimentally that the later is caused by a filterable virus and introduced a preventive inoculation.

EMIL VON BEHRING (1854-1917): His great discovery was in 1890 of the principle of "SERUM TREATMENT" and of "DIPTHERIA ANTISERUM with Von Behring there was SHIBASABURO KITASATO (1852-1931) a Japanis who was under Koch for six years. Though the "BACILLUS of PLAGUE" was discovered in 1894, the same was discovered independently at Hong Kong by a French Bacteriologist ALEXANDRE YERSIN.

Later on Behring and Kitasato discovered an antitoxin of "TETANUS". Behring from 1894 began to produce the Diptheria Antiscrum in large scale, as a recognised specific treatment for diptheria in man. The success of diptheria antitoxin led to many attempts to treat other specific infections by immane sera but except in Tetanus and serpent poisoning FERDINAND GUEPUE (1852) a Prussian army surgeon devoted his much times on important works on Fermentation (1883), Bacteriology of Milk (1884-1912), Chlorophyll (1887-1905), disinfects (1889-1891).

The work of the following persons led the epoch making discoveries in the bacteriology.

(a) FRIEDRICH LOEFFLER (1852-1915): Bacilins "Diptheria" and "Glander".

(b) RICHARD PFEIFFER (1958): Influenza Bacillus and microccus. Cataralis.

(c) ALBERT NEISSER (1855-1916): Gonoccus.

(d) ARMAUER HANSEN (!841-1912): Leprosy bacillus.

(e) SIR ALMORTH WRIGHT: Vaccine theraphy.

(f) SIR WILLIAM BOGG LEISHMANN: (1865-1926).

A simple method of staining the malarial parasite and original contribution on kalazar or DUM DUM FEVER known as leishmaniasis.

(g) SIR ALEXANDER OGSTON (1944-1929): First identified staphyloceus and differentiated it from streptoccus.

(h) THEOBALD SMITH (1859-1934): Anaphylaxis and differentiation of Human and Bovine Tabercalosis.

(l) JULES BORDET: A nobel prize winner of 1919. He discovered bacterial hemolysis and the specific bacillus of whooping cough. He was a great pioneer in the theory of serology and immunity reaction.

Three leading contributions to the study of syphilis in the early part of 19th century were made by three persons SPIROCHAETA PALLIDA, the causal orgaism of syphilis: (i) In 1905 FRITZ RICHARD SCHAUDDIN (1871-1906) of Hambrug discovered, (ii) In 1906 August VON WASSERMANN (1866-1925) of Berlin discovered the blood test for syphilis known as "washerman reaction" and in (iii) 1909 PAUL EHRLICH of Frankfut discovered No. 606 a remedy for syphilis know as "salvarsan" and later on 1912 a less tonic substance know as "Neo-Salvarsan".

Thus gradually with increased knowledge of cellular pathology and chemistry and molecular biology, bacteriology became a highly organised science of immense practical efficacy and opened a new era in sanitation as environmental and personal bacteriology.

(j) WILLIAM HENRY WELCH (1950-1934): In 1892 discovered the bacillus of gas gangrene (Bacillus aerogenes capsulatus).

(k) HOWARD TAYLOR RICKETTS (1871-1910)

He identified a micro-organism which was neither bacillus nor protozoa. They were known as Rickettsia infections which include trench fever conveyed by Louse, Japan fever by harvest mite and Rocky mountain fever by Tick.

(l) SIMON FLEXIVER (1863) discovered etiology of cerebrospinal meningitis -infentile pollio-encephalitis.

(m) VICRO CLARENCE VAUGHAN (1851-) In 1896 found the poison producing bacillus in ice-cream and cheese.

(n) PAUL EHRIGH (!854-1915) a German improved method of drying and fixing blood smear by heat. He discovered the mastcells and detection of their granulation by basic aniline staining-division of blood corpuscles into neutrophil, basophil and oxyphilic. He introduced Fuchsin stain for tuberculosis which was the basis of calling them as acid-fast and diazo-reaction of typhoid urine, sulpho-diazo-benzol test for Bilirubin, first antliner of "side chain theory".

(o) AUGUST VON WASSERMANN (1866-1926)

Hemolytic Diagosis of Syphilis. The original Wasserman reaction has followed by ingenious modification and checks as Flocculation reaction of Meincke (1911) and Vernes and many others.

OTOLOGY

Otology has been recognised as a separate branch of medicine from the 18th century. But the intricacies of arual anatomy attracted many anatomist of every generation. EUSTACHIUS and FALLOPIUS imprinted their names upon the organ of hearing from 16th century. EUSTACHIUS was a professor at Collegia della sapienza in Rome. In 1552 he completed his Tabulae Anatomicoe, a set of superb plates drawn by himself, which remained unprinted in papal library for 162 years. Finally pope Clement XI presented those engraved plates to his physician Lancisi who published them in 1714 with his own notes. The drawing were more accurate in delination than those of vesalius.

BARTOLOMEUS EUSTACHIUS (1520-74) discovered the EUSTACHIAN Tube the thoracic duct, the suprarenal bodies, and the abducens nerve, the origin of optic nerve, the Cochlea, the pulmonary views, the muscels of thorat at neck, the correct picture of the aterees. He wrote the best treatise of his time on the structure of the teeth giving the nerve and blood supply.

FALLOPIUS or GABRIELE Fallopices, (1523-62) was a loyal pupil of Versailles discovered and described the chorda tympain, the emicricular canals the sphenoid sinus, the ovaries and fallopian tube, the round ligaments, the trigeminal, auditory glossopharyngcal nerve and named the vagina and placenta.

But the first monograph containing the diseases of the ear was "TRAITE DE L'OUIC" a little book by J.G. DUVERNEY (1648-1730) a professor of Anatomy in Paris.

Another name familiar to every otologist is ANTONIO VALSALVA (1666-1723). whose "TRACTATUS DE AURE HU-MANA was published at Bologna in 1704. The treatment of deafness by "Valsalva" a method of inflation, which was carried as step further GUYOT, a french a Postmaster of Versailles invented the Eustachian Catheter and used it to release his own deafness.

Among the contribution of Capital importance in the studies of Structure and, Physiology of the ear were not only Valsalva but SCARPA (1772-89) and COTUGNO (1774) and the morphological essay of GEOFFROY (1778) and COMPARETTI (!789).

The existence of an elastic fluid in the labyrinth and its role in the transmission of sound was noted even before coliegno by THEODOR PYL in 1742.

Catheterization was first attempted by the post master GUYOT in 1724 but subsequently performed by ARCHIBALD CLELAND in 1741. ELI a reputed quack is credited with first to note perforation of the tympanic membrane for deafness.

In 1755 JOHNATHAN WATHEN had treated catarrhal deafness by means of injection into the Eustachian tube through a catheter inserted into the nose.

The most important in the history of surgery is the opening of mastoid process for the first time by JEAN-LOUIS PETIT in 1736.

Later on many such operations were performed by a Prussian army surgeon JASSER in 1776 and by J.G.H. FIELITZ, A.F.L. OFFLER and the Danish Surgeon ALEXANDER KOLPIN IN 1796.

Various attempts were made by many people to establish otology on scientific basis and JOHN CUNNINGHAM SAUNDERS who also practice opthalmology founded in 1805 the "handen dispensary for curing diseases of the Eye and Ears" which was ultimately turned as "Royal opthalmic Hospital.

The first treatise on diseases of the ears was written by JEAN-ITARD a military surgeon of Paris (1775-1838) in 1821 and later important books were written by Joseph Toynbee (1860), Anton Friedrich Von Troltsch (1866), Lawrence Turnbull (1872). Sir William. B. Dalby (1873), St. John Roosa (1873), Adam Politzer Victor Urbantschitsch.

Important contributions were made by MAX SCHULTZE who described the nerve ending in the labyrinth (1858), HELMHOLIZ the mechanies of the ossicles and tympanic membrane, GOLTZ the physiological significance of the semicurlar canals.

ADAM POLITZER (1835-1920) of Alberti Hungary, was first to obtain picture of the tympanic membrane by illumination (1865) which he afterward illustrated in an atlas of 14 plates and 392 pictures.

The transmission of sounds through the cranial bones in diagnosis of aural diseases was first studied by JOHANN C.A. LUCAE (1870) and great advances were made in this regard was made by FRIEDRICH BEZOLD and also by TAUBER in 1877 who gave the first description of mastoiditis and introduced new tests for audition in deaf mutism and in unilateral deafness.

Among the other advances were the Weber and Rinne tests, Hartmann's diapasons and Sir Francis Galton's whistle for determining the superior limits of audation.

The most important works in surgery of the ear in the 19th century were made by SIR ASTLEY COOPER (1801), SIR WILLIAM WILDE (1843-63) and by JAMES HINTON (1827-1975).

HINTON was a as a Philosopher and his little book on the "The mystery of pain" is still read. In 1873 HERMANN SCHWARTZE and ADOLPH EYSELL described the method of opening the mastoid by chiseling. The two other EMANUEL ZAUFAL (1884) and ERNST KUSTER made good improvement in the mastoid Surgery.

In 1890 LUDWIG STACKE introduced excision of the ossicles. In 1861 the aural vertigo was first described by PROSPER MENIERE (1799-1862) This was verified by CHARCOT.

The relation between nystagmus and vestinuelar or care bellar disease was noted by PURKINJE and FLOWRENS, which was further developed by ROBERT BARANY. In 1906 Rebert Barany cleared up the hazy subject of aural vertigo or the Menieres diseases, especially in differentiating it from allied or adjacent lesions in carebellum from epilepsy or from ordinary nystagmus.

Labyrinthine vertigo or "vestibular nystagmus" is interpreted by

Barany as a disturbance of function of the vestibular nerve or the organs to which it is different causes with which it might be confused. He has introduced a number of ingenious differential tests, such as production of nystagmus by irrigation of the external meatus with cold or warm water (caloric test) or by having a patient try to point at an object with his eyes shut after having previously touched it (static test) and he has been able to prove his case by successful operations on the cerebellum or the internal ear. He has also devised a "Noise Machine" for testing paracusis Willisii, and other diagnostic novelties will be incomplete if we do not mention the name of ADAM POLITZER (1835-1920) who did much to upkeep the speciality of this subject.

His interest was noted by his publication "GESCHICHTE DER OHRENHEIL KUNDE" in 1913 before his death, a masterpiece of historical research.

Modern oto-rhio-larygology has much improved by inventions of improved instruments such as Electric audiometer and larygoscope in 1855 by MANUEL GARCIA who was really a singing master of Paris. Laryngology continued it advances in Vienna under the well known OTTO CHIARI (1853-1918) and MARKUS HAJEK (!861-1941).

In Britian SIR MORELL MACKENZIE was a reputed man in this field with sell reputation and had the opportunity of attending the German Emperor Frederick III the historic case of cancer on the larynx.

Laryngology and rhinology were specially advanced by the introduction of larynogoscopy by Benjamin Babington (1829), Robert Liston (1837), Manuel Garcia (1855), Ludwing Turck (1858-60) and Johann Czermak (1858) of rhinoscopy by Philip Bozzmi (1773-1809) in 1807 and successfully by Czermak (1850) of authoscopy of the larynz and trachea without the mirror by Alfred Kirstein (1860-), Mainz (1898) and of direct bronchoscopy by Gustay Killian (1850-1921) of Karakowizer of Vienna who was the first physician in America to demonstrate the vocal cords. In 1858 also Ephraim Cutter of Massachusetts devised a laryngoscope (Schwebelaryngoskopie) was introduced by Killian (1912). The anatomy of the larynx and the physiology of the voice and speach were investigated by Jhoannes Muller (1839), Ernst von Brucke (1856), F.C. Donders (1870), Hubert von luschka(1872) and Carl Merkel (Authropohonik, 1876). Max Schultze investigated the histology and nerve-endings of the Schneiderian membrance (1863), Emil Zucker-kandl (1861-1921), the anatomy and pathology of the accessory sinuses (1862-92) and Hemdrik Zwaardemaker (1857), the physiology of smell (1895). A perfected method of photographing the larynx was devised by Thomas Rushmore French (1884). Important early treatises on laryngology were those of John Cheyne (1777-1836) on the pathology of the membrance of the laryox and Brouchia (1809). William Henry Porter (1790-1861) on the surgical pathology of the larynx and trachca (!826). Armed Trousseau and Hipplyte Belloc on laryngeal phthisis, chronic laryngitis, and disorders of the voice (1837), Horace Green (1802-66) on diseases of the air passages (1846) Samuel D Gross on foreign bodies in the air passages (1854) and Sir Morell Mackenzie on laryngeal tumours (1871). As Bryson Delavan says: The sciences of laryngology and rhinology were placed upon a firm literary basis through the three treatises of J. Sol is (cohen (1872), Sir Morell Mackenzie (1880) and Francke Huntington Bosworth (1881-91) in 1856-1868, In tubation of the laryux was first done in Paris in connection with tracheotomy by Trousseau (1851-1859), and perfected through the conscientious labors (1885-1888) of the self sacrificing of Behring from 1894 began to produce the Diptheria Antiscrum in large scale, as a recognised specific treatment for diptheria in man. The success of diptheria antitoxin led to many attempts to treat other specific infections by immane sera but except in Tetanus and serpent poisoning Joseph P.O. Dwyer (1811-98) of Cleveland, Ohio, whose name stands with those of Semmelweis and Crede as one of the great benefactors infact life. Horace Green (1802-1866) of Crittenden. Vermont a friend of Trousseau, was the pioneer of larynoglogy and was first to treat the throat by local application (1838) the first to describe cystic and malignant laryngeal growths (1851-1852) and the author of important works on croup. Elsberg, J. Solis Cohen, Knight, and Lefferts founded the Archires of Laryngology (New York 1880-1883). As to instrumentation, the ancient Icelanders used a ring knife uvulotome, the tonsillotome was invented by P.S. Physick (1828), the ring-knife tonsillotome by Fthnestock (1832), Charles Henrl Ehrmann (1792-1878) was the first to remove a laryngeal polyp. (1844), Victor von Bruns (1812-13) first enucleated a laryngeal polyp by the bloodless method (1862) and was the pioneer of Laryngoscopic surgery (!865). Rudolph Voltolini (1819-89) first employed the galvanocautery in larungeal surgery (1865) and performed the first laryngeal operation through the mouth with external illumination (1889) paralysis of the vocal cord was carefully studied by CARI-GERARDT in 1863-72. Role of the Recurrent laryngeal nerve in complete and incomplete were studied by OTTO-MAR ROSENBACH (1880) and later on by SIR FELIX SIMMCN.

LUDWING GRUNWALF made a good attempt for the surgical treatment of Nasal supperation and diseases of Ethmoid and sphencid. There were many who contributed in the field of diseases of more in the 20th and 21th centuries and the advancement is still continuing with more instruments.

AUSCULTATION

For clinical purpose the use of Stethoscope was really an advancement.

A French named as RENE THEOPHILE HYACINTHE LAENNEC (1781-1826) though he was a physician of distinct he could not proceed much because of his health. He was attacked with Tuberculosis that was one of the causes of his early death at the age of 45 years.

At one time of his medical career he was appointed as a physician at Necker Hospital.

He died at the age of 45 years. Shortly after his appointment as physician to the Necker Hospital in 1816 he had occasion to examine a patient whose stoutness made it difficult for the Physician to hear the heart sounds. Inspired, it is said by having noticed two children playing with a log of wood, one tapping or scraping it while the other listened by holding his ear against the sawn end, Laennec rolled a quire of paper into a cylinder, and placing one end on the patient's chest and the other to his own ear, discovered that he could hear the heart's action, "In a manner more clear and distinct than I had ever been able to do by the immediate application of the ear." Auscultation by the direct application of the ear to the chest of the patient has been long known in medicine, and even. Hippocrates had described the "Creaking as of leather", which is audible in pleursy. But as Laennec stated, "the older method was not only ineffective but inconvenient, indelicate, and in hospitals even disgusting," The stethoscope described by Laennec in his book, Traite do I Auscultation mediate (1818), was "a cylinder of wood an inch and a half in diameter and a foot long, perforated by a bore three lines wide and hollowed out into funnel shape at one of its extremities". The labour necessary to perfect his discovery and to compose his treatise was nearly fatal to the author, and he was obliged to retire to Brittany to recuperate.

The work created a sensation in Paris, and was well received in other countries, as Laennec not only described the sounds heard by the stethoscope, coining new terms such as pectoriloguy, aegophony, crepitations, rhonchi, but in the second edition he added a detailed account of the diseases of the chest as then known, making his book of permanent value. He liberally acknowledges the labours of others, mentioning, for example, that "the employment of the new method must not make us forget that of Auenbrugger".

Laennec was the originator of certain term like "egophony" pectoilquy" the sonorus and sibilant racles.

Leopold Auen Brugger (1722-1809) was the son of an innkeeper of Garz and he had often used PERCUSSION to ascertain the level of wine in his father's Casks. This principle he applied to the human chest when he became physician in the military hospital of Vienna. The process of Auscultation in diseases of chest and heart is related with the use of Stethoscope. In this regard the contribution of the eminent physician of Iris medical School-WILLAM STOKE (1804-1878) is a matter of great events Stoke was educated in Edintrergh in 1825 and while only twenty one he publised a small treatise on the stethoscope inspired on the study by Laennec's book in 1837 and 1845. He wrote two books namely, "The diagnosis and treatment of Diseases of the chest" and "Diseases of Heart and aorta".

He gave much stress on the physical signs in valvular diseases of the heart and that the condition of the heart muscles was of much importance than the state of the valve which was also by Sir James Mackenzie.

Along with Cheyne, he described a type of in serious heart diseases known as "CHEYNE-STOKE RESPIRATION. He also recorded a slow pulse with syncopal attack, named as "STOKE ADAMS SYNDROME" with ROBERT ADAMS.

Another name in the History of medicine JOSEF SKODA (1805-81) of New School for his contrbution in matters of percussion and Auscultation.

His principal contribution to medicine was his treatise on Auscultation and percussion (1839) in which he tried to classify the different sounds so heard during percussion and auscultation in the chest which ranged according to musical pitch and tonasity and alternating from dull to hollow, clear to dull, Tympanitic to muftled, high to deep.

"SKODA'S RESONACE" the drum like sound heart in pneumonia and precardial effusion is a permanent aid in modern diagnosis given in memory of Skoda.

The Physics of sound was not well knows during Skoda's time it was because of his acoustic experience that made the medical diagnosis into proper descriptive term than the loose term that were used by the French physicians.

In 1890 an important treatise on "Auscultation and percussion was published by CARL GERHARDT (1833-1902), a professor at Jena Wurzburg and Berline.

Lastly we must pay respect to AUSTIN FLINT SR (1812-95) and HENRY IN GERSOLL BOWDITCH (1808-92) for their contribution and treatise on "Auscultation and Percussion" and STETHOSCOPE".

INDEX

A.V. Graefe	117
Abernethy	66
Abu Mansur	11
Act of 1540	32
Adam Politzer	132
Adam Politzer	133
Al Mansur	12
Albrecht Von Haller	55
Albucasis	10
Alcmaeon	19
Alexandria Roman	25
Alfred Karl Graefi	119
Aliis Inserviendo Consumor	43
Allvar Gulistran	122
Almal Ki	10
Ambroise Pare	30
Anaesthetic Properties	103
Anatomy Teacher	15
Andreas Vasalius	28
Andre Levert	63
Anima	50
Antenatal	106
Anthanasius Kircher	43
Antiseptics	107
Antiseptic	58
Antoine Lauren Zavoisier	78
Antonio Valsalva	131
Antonio Valsalv	41
Antonj Van Leeuwenhoek	43
Anti Diphtheritic Serum	128
Aqueduct	30
Arctaeus	26
Aristotle	24
Aristotle	24
Aristotle Contributions	24
Arnold of Villanova	14

Asclepiades	25
Astely Cooper	66
Asthenic	25
Atreya	9
Austin Flint Sr	136
Avenzoar	11
Ayur-veda	6
Babylonian medical ethics	4
Bacteriology	123
Bartholin	43
Bartholomeus Anglicus	13
Batrolomeus Eustachius	30
Bell's Paralysis	82
Bernard De Gordom	14
Blood-Letting	48
Blood Pressure	78
Broussais	25
Brunner	43
C.G.Ehrenberg	124
Carbolic Acid	110
Cartesian	39
Carl Wernicke	96
Carl Ernst Von Baer	83
Carl Gerhardt	136
Carl Ludwig	84
Carl Rokitansky	124
Catgut	111
Celsus	26
Cell Theory	85
Jacob Henle	87
Chang Chung King	18
Charaka	6
Charles Mc Burney	113
Cheyne-Stoke Respiration	136
Chinese	18
Chinese herb Mahuang	18
Chinese medicine	4
Chloroform	105
Christoph Scheiner	114
Chrle of Willis	46

Corvisart	75
Crawford Long	104
Daniel Drake	91
De Subtilitate	34
Dioscorides	25
Dioscorides	24
Dr. F.C.S. Hahnemann	51
Dr. James Young Simpson	105
Dr. John Fother Gill	72
Dr. John Howard	72
Dr. John Snow	105
Dr. Robert Liston	105
Dr. William Tuke	72
Dr.Jacob Henle	82
Dr.John Caius	37
Edmund Chapman	59
Edmud Chapmal	62
Edme Mariotte	114
Edward Jenner	71
Edward Jenner	66
Egyptian medicine	4
Eighteenth Century Medicine	49
Emil Du Bois Reymond	84
Emil Kraepelin	96
Empedocies	19
Ephraim Mc Dowell	91
Erasistratus	25
Ernst Von Bergmann	112
Ether Anaesthesia	105
Ether Frolic	104
Extractor or Forceps	59
Ferdinand Jullius	125
First Known Medical Men	4
First Medical Book Printed	26
Fissure of Sylvius	43
Fracastorius	35
Franciscan Roger Bacon	14
Francis Bacon	37
Francis De La Boe or Sylvius	43
Francis Glisson	46

Francois Xavier Bichat	69
Franz Anton Mesmer	79
Freud	100
Friedrich Bezold	132
Friedrich Hoffman	50
Gabriel Fallopius	30
Galen	26
Galileo Galilei	39
Gardner Colton	104
Gaspare Tagliacozzi	32
Gaspare Aselli of Cremona	40
Geber	12
Georg Ernst Stahl	50
Geschichte Der Ohrenheil Kunde	133
Giovanni	69
Giovani Alphonso Borelli	45
Giorgio Baglivi	45
Govert Bidloo	43
Greece and Roman medicine	4
Guido Lanfranchi	14
Guy De Chauliac	16
Guyde Chauliac	17
Volkhava or Walfaman	17
Gynaecology	113
Haly Ben Abbas	10
Haly Ben Abbas	13
Hendrik Van Deventer	45
Henry Grey	83
Henry in Gersoll Bowditch	136
Henry Jacob Bigelow	112
Heri de Mondeville	16
Hermann Boerhaave	53
Hermann Boer Haave	114
Hermann Von Helmholtz	83
Herophilus	25
Hertzian Waves	84
Hieronymus Fracastorius Girolamo	35
Hindeyo Noguchi	19
Hippocrates	19
Hippocrates	6

Hippocratic Facies	23
Homoeopathy	52
Howard Taylor Ricketts	130
Hon Robert Boyle	41
Huatu	18
Hugh Crichton Miller	97
Hutchinson's Facies	112
Hutchinson's Mask	112
Hutchison's Triad	112
Hwangt	18
Iatro-Chemical	45
Iatro-Mechanical	45
Iatro-Physical	45
Iatro-Physicists	39
Ibn Al Haitham	10
Ibn Sina	10
Imhotep	6
India's ancient medicine	4
Inoculated with Syphilis	128
Inoculation houses	70
Jabu	12
Jacques Daviel	115
James Currie	74
Japan	18
Jan Swammerdam	43
Jean-Itard	132
Jean Nicholas	74
Jean Palfyn	62
Jerome Cardan	34
Jewish medicine	4
Johannes Muller	83
Johann C.A. Lucae	132
Johathan Wathen	131
Johm Cheyne	90
Johnmayow	42
John Condlly	95
John Abernethy	67
Antonio Scarpa	67
Antonio	68
John Brown	51

John Conolly	95
John Cunningham Saunders	131
John Floyer	74
John Fothergill	73
John Howard	73
John Hughlings Jackson	122
John Hunter	64
John Hunter	63
John Huxman	59
John Radicliffe	73
John Woodall	59
Joseph Desault	68
Joseph Barthez of Montpellier	50
Joseph Black	79
Joseph Clover	105
Joseph Clover	106
Joseph Hyrtl	83
Joseph Lister	107
Joseph Meister	126
Joseph Priestley	79
Josef Skoda	90
Lead Colic	59
Leonardo Da Vinci	28
Leopold Auenbrugger	74
Lucas Championniere	111
Ludwing Grunwalf	134
Ludwig Stacke	132
Lyden	43
Magic Man	4
Maitre-Jan	115
Man-Midwife	59
Mandragora	8
Manuel Garcia	133
Marcello Malpighi	41
Marion Sims	92
Marie Sklodowska Curie	93
Marshall Hall	85
Mathew Baillie	70
Mayow	41
Medical Act of 1958	32

Medical Papyri	5
Metal Blades Forcep	62
Miasmata	127
Michael Farady	104
Michael Scot	104
Mithridaticum and Theriac	25
Mondino De Luzzi	16
Montpellier	14
Morphological classification of bacteria	125
Neiching	18
Niels Rybero Finsen	93
Nitrous Oxide	104
Nitrous Oxide	106
Oath of Hippocratic	21
Obstetric Forcep	113
Obstetric Forcep	62
Opothalmoscope	84
Opthalmology	113
Opthalmometer	114
Otology	130
Bartolomeus Eustachius	131
Otto Friedrik Muller	124
Pacchioni	43
Paracelsus	32
Paris Albert Von Bolstaot	15
Paul Broca	83
Paul Ehrigh	130
Paul Reclus	111
Pen Tsoas	18
Percival Pott	63
Percussion	135
Peter Lowe	32
First English Text Book on Surgery	32
Peter Chamberlen	62
Peter Smith	105
Peyer	43
Philippus Aureolus Theophrastus Bobbastus Von Hohnheim	32
Philippe Pinel	95
Pierre Franco	30
Piere Briston	49

Pietro-D-A-Rgelata	17
Plantarum	24
Pneuma	26
Pollender	127
Pre Historic Era	1
Preventive Medicine	106
Psychiatry	95
Public Health	76
Pythagoras	19
Rademacher and Hahnemann	34
Radiology	92
Radium	112
Rcnald	16
Recurrent Laryngeal Nerve	27
Regnier De Graaf	43
Rene Descartes	114
Rene Descartes	38
Respiration Oxygen	78
Red Cross	58
Rhazes	10
Richard Bright	87
Richard Gwoers	122
Richard Lower of Cornwall	41
Richard Mead	73
Robert Craves	90
Robert Henry Elliot	123
Robert Hooke	43
Robert Koch	124
Robert Liston	107
Robert Whytt	57
Roentgen	81
Roger	16
Roger	16
Royal College of Physician	37
Rudolf Virchow	124
Sacteya	9
Saint Erasmus	12
Saint Apollonia	12
Saint Bernardine	12
Saint Blaise	12

Saint Lawrence	12
Samuel David	113
Sanctorius	45
Sanitary Hygiene	78
Sarah Nelmes	71
Scheiner	114
School of Salero	12
Sero-Diagnostic test for typhoid fever	128
Shen Nung	18
Simon Flexiver	130
Sims	92
Sir Charles Bell	81
Sir Fielding Ould	59
Sir Humphry Davy	104
Sir Issac Newton	49
Sir James Paget	112
Sir John Pringle	57
Sir Jonathan Hutchison	112
Howard Kelly	112
Sir Morell Mackenzie	133
Sir Richard Manningham	59
Sir Thomas Smith Clouston	96
Skoda's Resonace	136
Spirochaeta Pallida	129
Steam Sterilization	112
Stensen	43
Stephen Jenner	71
Stethoscope	76
Sthenic	25
Stock Adams Syndrome	136
Sumerian	4
Susruta	6
Syphilis	35
Tabula Anatomicae	29
Tartagta	34
Tean Louis Petit	68
Theodore Kocher	112
Theodore Turquet	46
Theophile Hyacinthe Laennec	76
Theophrastus	24

Theophrastus	24
Thomas Vicary	30
Thomas Dimsdale	70
Thomas Addison	89
Thomas Linacre	37
Thomas Phayre	37
Thomas Smith Clouston	97
Thomas Sydenham	47
Thomas Willis	46
Thomas Young	115
Thomas Young	84
The Cowpox	72
Torcular Herophili	25
Treatise of Midwifery	59
Treatise on Scurvy	58
Tubercle bacillus	127
Tuberculin	127
Twelfth & Thirteenth Century	13
Typhus	36
Usei Bia	10
Vicro Clarence	130
Vieuwssens	43
Virchow	124
Virus of Cholera	127
Vis Medicatris Naturae	24
Vital Principle	27
Vital Principle	50
Von Helmholtz	116
Warton	43
Wilhelm Griesinger	95
William Clowes	32
William Cheselden	63
William Cullen	53
William Giffard	59
William Harvey	39
William Heberden	73
William Henry	130
William Hewson	66
William Hunter	54
William Hyde Wollaston	116

William Keen	113
William Sharpey	85
William Smellie	59
William Smellie	62
William Stokes	90
William Stoke	136
William Withering	74
Wirsung	43
Wooden Forcep	62
Zacharias Jansen	43
Zacharias Jansen Microscope	42